I SEE ADDICTION

"It takes an addict to help an addict."

"For the first time in my life, I am happy without an asterisk next to the word 'happy.'"

"Heavenly Father changed me on the inside when I was unable to change myself."

"When I say I am an addict in recovery, the emphasis is on *recovery*. It means that I no longer act out on my addiction—at all—ever."

"This is where I always wanted to be."

"Heavenly Father promises shelter and rest to those who seek Him. He hasn't let me down."

"We want other people to have what we have—or simply to know that it is even possible. We want to see LDS husbands and wives with confidence in each other. We want to see Latter-day Saint women who trust their husbands, who don't cry themselves to sleep at night, who don't wonder what happened to their 'happily ever after.'

"We want to see Mormon men worthy of the priesthood they bear, worthy to lay their hands on their children's heads and utter blessings that are too wonderful to describe, worthy to attend the temple with their wives and feel the presence of angels, worthy to stand as disciples of Christ having felt the full redemptive power of His Atonement. We want to see our people enjoying peace and love in this life with no secrets gnawing away at their insides."

RECOVERY IS POSSIBLE AND IT IS WONDERFUL!

RowboatAndMarbles.org

Sitting in a Rowboat Throwing Marbles at a Battleship

Essays of Hope about Recovery from Sex and Pornography Addiction from the LDS Perspective

Andrew Pipanne

Disclaimer: The author of this book is an addict working on his own recovery. He is not a trained medical doctor, psychiatric professional or therapist. All opinions expressed herein are those of the author and do not reflect the policy or doctrinal position of any church including The Church of Jesus Christ of Latter-day Saints. Readers are encouraged to seek out and rely upon the counsel of trained professionals in dealing with sex and pornography addiction and all that goes with it.

© 2011-12 Andrew Pipanne. All rights reserved. Printed in the United States of America.

ISBN 978-0-9858669-0-7

Table of Contents

Acknowledgments . . . . *vii*

Introduction . . . . *ix*

1. Sitting in a Rowboat Throwing Marbles at a Battleship: A personal story of recovery from sex and pornography addiction *1*

2. A Letter to LDS Wives: What every Mormon woman needs to know about sex and pornography addiction *13*

3. The ABCs of Porn Addiction: The real reasons why so many LDS men can't kick the pornography problem *25*

4. Porn Addiction Is Like a Muck Fire in My Brain: Why merely stopping the porn binging isn't enough *47*

5. Another Letter to the Wife Who Suffers in Silence Because of Her Husband's Porn Addiction: How LDS women can know if their husbands are sexually sober—and what to do if they're not *57*

6. Getting on the Same Page: 12 changes Mormons should make right now to their thinking about sex and pornography addiction . . . *63*

7. A Letter to Theo: Moral agency and why a sponsor is vital to an addict's recovery *73*

8. The Silent 70 Percent: Seeing the sex and pornography crisis among Latter-day Saints as it really is *77*

9. Is Recovery from Sex and Pornography Addiction Even Possible? The short answer is a resounding YES! *93*

10. This Is What Recovery Feels Like! Ever wonder what goes on in the mind of a recovering sex addict? Read this! *97*

Acknowledgments

I OWE A HUGE DEBT of gratitude to the many individuals who were directly and indirectly involved in the writing of this book. Thanks to the men of Sexaholics Anonymous who have befriended, supported and encouraged me in my recovery. Thanks for showing me what unconditional love looks like, sounds like and feels like. Thanks for teaching me patience and forgiveness. Thank you for allowing me to see how the Master has changed your lives and made you into new men. Thanks most of all for telling me and then demonstrating to me that recovery is possible and fabulous.

Thanks to my sponsors, men of God with hearts of gold and the wisdom of Solomon. You have reminded me that so much of the good in the world emanates from Rome—not all of it comes from Salt Lake City.

Thanks also to those I have sponsored. I hope that I have been able to teach you just a fraction of what you have taught me. Thanks especially to the guys who have stuck with it, confirming to me that honesty, humility and hard work lead to sobriety, serenity and lasting recovery.

My wife and I will be forever grateful to our friends C.T. and G.T. Thanks for fighting for us, for being there for us, and for being patient with us. We apologize for being such high-maintenance friends. We can't imagine the last thirteen years without you and your family.

Likewise, we lack words to express our love for J. and J. for saving us. It's evident that God put you in our lives 20 years ago with the year 2010 clearly on His mind. Thank you for walking the path ahead of us and for being ready to share your experience, strength and hope so we could begin our recovery after two days instead of two years.

I express thanks to N.S., an inspired and inspiring counselor. Thanks for patiently and gently taking me to the parts of my mind, life and history that I had spent a lifetime trying to forget, all so that I could find understanding, forgiveness and healing.

I regret that Roy K. passed away before I had a chance to shake his hand and tell him thanks. In answer to his favorite question, "Where's the sobriety?" I would have told him with an enthusiastic smile, "It's right here!"

Thanks to Paul the Apostle, who told me to grow up and be a man. "When I was a child, I spake as a child, I understood as a child, I thought as a child: but when I became a man, I put away childish things." I think that I have finally begun to put away those childish things that kept me from understanding the addiction that was killing me.

To my kids, I express my love and gratitude by way of living amends. I now hope to be the father you always needed me to be.

Lastly, my love to Claire. Thanks for staying. Thanks for doing hard things. No man has ever loved a woman as much as I love you. You are more important to me than breathing!

Introduction

I AM A RECOVERING sex and pornography addict. When I say I am an addict in recovery, the emphasis is on *recovery*. It means that I no longer act out on my addiction—at all—ever. Through involvement in a recovery process including therapy and 12-Step meetings, I've regained the ability to make choices. That's the miracle of recovery from addiction—once again being able to make choices. Heavenly Father promises shelter and rest to those who seek Him. He hasn't let me down.

There are several reasons for which this book came into being. When I first began writing these essays, I wanted to record the miracle of my recovery from addiction. The healing experiences were coming so quickly and with such force that I had begun to panic at the thought that no one around me could possibly know all of what I was going through. I had to write down as much as I could.

I wanted my wife to understand what I had learned: not only that complete and lasting recovery was indeed possible, but also why recovery was possible this time around—after the ten million failures that had preceded it. I also wanted my bishop and stake president to read the details of a repentance and recovery experience made possible because the sinner was finally able to truly forsake the sin. In addition, I wanted my wife's family to know what we knew so they wouldn't think she was crazy for staying. That's how it started.

As my ideas and understanding of true recovery evolved, I began to seek out other LDS men whose experiences mirrored my own, who had finally found sexual sobriety and recovery from addiction, and who were looking to share it. To my dismay, I couldn't find very many. Most of the forums and blogs out there seemed to recount stories of failed recovery from the viewpoint of the devastated wife. The pain was plentiful; the hope was scarce.

The few men who did venture to share their "recovery" experiences made it clear by their vagueness and self-absorption that "recovery" for them meant binging or "slipping up" less often now than they had in the past. Although they were still acting out, they seemed to be suggesting to everyone that this was "as good as it gets," something I knew from my own experience to be false, misleading and frankly self-serving to the active addict. They were effectively grooming shockingly low expectations in their wives and others. Someone had to take a stand and say that periodic binging on porn and masturbation is *not* sobriety and that those who binge are *not* in recovery.

The lone voice of true sobriety calling from the wilderness was Steven Croshaw at *SALifeline.org*. Steven and his wife Rhyll courageously went public to tell their story of redemption, recovery and forgiveness with an emphasis on complete and lasting sobriety. Steven was kind enough to read many of my essays and assure me that they added value to the effort to educate the LDS population about *real* recovery from sex and pornography addiction. Steven also reminded me repeatedly to bridle my usually sharp tongue so as not to muddy up the message with my unresolved resentments.

The grand question that eventually loomed in my mind was: Why weren't more of the LDS men who were in complete recovery sharing their experience, strength and hope with those who were still suffering? I finally concluded (with feelings approaching despair) that we don't hear from very many of these guys because there simply *aren't* very many of them. Those Latter-day Saint men who were at one time acting out with porn and masturbation several times a week and have now succeeded in reducing their binging to once every three to six months are relatively pleased with their progress. Still, they don't want to go shouting *that* story from the rooftops. I don't blame them. I wouldn't either.

My personal experiences with the Church's Pornography Addiction Support Group (PASG) suggested to me that too many LDS men simply did not know that it's even possible to stop completely and permanently the binging on porn and masturbation. Often, the men with whom I interacted at those meetings seemed resigned to a life of white-knuckle struggling against the compulsions, accompanied from time to time by the inevitable "slips."

Other LDS men who also have achieved *long-term recovery* have since recounted to me similar experiences with PASG. The hopeful message of complete sobriety and true recovery simply was not getting out there to those who most needed to hear it. I wanted to change that.

The latest questions for me have been: How can I best explain the roots of addiction in a simple way so that Latter-day Saints can quickly see and understand that this is not just a "little problem"? How can I help Latter-day Saints understand that addiction cannot be overcome *in isolation*? How can I help Latter-day Saint members and leaders realize that the LDS men and women out there in *long-term recovery* from their addiction are hands-down the best resource to help those now suffering in silence?

Further, how can I can encourage Latter-day Saints to learn from the recovering addicts how to stop the binging once and for all, and how to stand up and be the men God intended them to be, the men their wives wish they were, and the men their children think they are? How can I instill in both men and women who struggle a hope that they can regain their integrity and actually soon be happier than they have ever been? How can I help spouses understand that this is not their fault, they didn't cause it, and they can't cure or even control their addicts' sickness? How can I promise hope for complete recovery to those individuals who become willing to do *whatever it takes*? These essays contain the answers I found to those questions. They talk about doing *whatever it takes* because

Recovery is possible and it is wonderful!

Note: Most of the essays in this compilation were originally written so they could each be read and understood independently of the others. For this reason, there is some occasional overlap and repetition of material.

Also note: As will be evident, this is not a book specifically about the Atonement of Jesus Christ. I believe in the Atonement. It is at the core of my faith and recovery. I have repeatedly experienced the healing balm of the Atonement in my life. Nevertheless, there are so many other voices out there infinitely more authoritative on that topic than mine. This book simply recounts how I was finally able to recover from the addiction that was destroying me, forsake the sin that was damning me, and at long last kneel before the Lord to ask for forgiveness, knowing that I now had the solution that would allow me never to be dragged back down into the hell of my addiction again. I believe it is one of the beautiful conundrums of the Gospel that Heavenly Father had to heal me first before he could forgive me.

A.P.

RowboatAndMarbles.org

1. Sitting in a Rowboat Throwing Marbles at a Battleship

A personal story of recovery from sex and pornography addiction

MY FIRST EXPERIENCE with pornography was at age six. Six-year-olds don't have the strength or capacity to say no to an older person looking to expose them to pornography. I certainly didn't. This was especially true after I heard the enticing description of the pictures I would find in the magazine hidden out in the cherry orchard. This older person, a teenage boy in the neighborhood where my family had recently moved, understood that the pornography he showed me became a secret we shared. He formed a covert bond with me and then used that bond to coax me to an isolated place so he could molest me. These experiences, coupled with an increasingly compulsive desire to flee into fantasy to escape the difficulty of living with a mentally ill parent, flipped a switch in me at a young age and I became a sex addict.

I think a lot of people have a pretty hazy idea of what a sex addict looks like. We imagine a pudgy, middle-aged guy in a trench coat with greasy hair and twitching, crazy eyes who sneaks around and peeps at women through their bedroom windows because he can't control his sex urges. The reality, however, is that in much the same way that there is a broad spectrum of alcoholics—from apparently able and functioning members of society at one extreme to the poor inebriate passed out in the gutter in some large city at the other—there is a broad spectrum of sex addicts.

To be sure, some sex addicts do sit in dark, dingy bedrooms with the curtains drawn surfing for porn on the internet for days at a time. But sex addicts are also very often some of the ordinary men, women, and children in the community around us. Some of them are your bosses or employees at work. Some of them are the people sitting with their families in front of you in the benches at church. Some of them are the kids on your child's baseball team. Although they come from all walks of life, I feel certain that most sex addicts share some common traits: First, they are miserable. Second, they wish that sex wasn't such an overwhelming part of their lives that devoured everything else. Third, I would also bet that many, if not most, sex addicts don't know that they are addicts. They think they just have a "little problem."

Addiction has been, and remains, very misunderstood. A lot of people fear that if we acknowledge that addiction is something beyond a particular person's control, we somehow give that individual a free pass to do whatever he wants in society without any accountability for the consequences. Although we *appear* to accept the reality of alcohol addiction, hard drug addiction, gambling addiction, a myriad of food addictions, and even shopping addiction, many of us honestly believe that addicts merely suffer from a deficiency of moral character. Addicts are not as righteous, are not as spiritual, are not as noble, and are not as sincere as the rest of us.

Addicts, we believe, just don't want to get out of their addiction. If addicts were truly serious and wanted to change, they would just stop doing what they're doing. Simply put, we think that addicts prefer to be the addicts that they are. They like the bondage of addiction, we assume, better than they like the freedom that the rest of us enjoy. Apparently, they choose addiction. I absolutely disagree.

The greatest misunderstanding about sex and pornography addiction, I believe, has to do with its size and power. I hope no one seriously thinks that an addiction is like a little red devil who sits on your shoulder whispering naughty thoughts in your ear and who may be easily disposed of by a flick of the finger. That might be a bad habit, but it's certainly not addiction.

Too many members of the LDS Church think that we're engaged in a fair fight with an evenly-matched opponent. Some Latter-day Saints probably imagine a couple wrestlers in a ring. Sometimes one wrestler (the addict) wins a round and sometimes the other one (the addiction) wins. The idea they have is that the addict just has to learn some moves, build some strength, think positively, listen to his coach, and eventually he will prevail over the addiction because he is the stronger wrestler. It's tough work, but that *evenly-matched* addiction can be whipped if the addict just becomes *stronger* than the addiction. While I certainly believe that addiction can be whipped, I completely disagree with any notion of a fair fight.

I see addiction in a much different way. I see a six-year-old boy in a tiny rowboat in the middle of the ocean with a handful of marbles. A grey, armored battleship is steaming towards him. He can hear it coming, but he can't see it very well because thick fog hangs everywhere. He is trying to sink the battleship by throwing marbles at it.

I am the six-year-old boy. My sex addiction is the battleship. Those marbles are my efforts to overcome the addiction *on my own*. The fog is misinformation, confusion, bias and judgmental attitudes about addiction. It keeps me from seeing two stark realities: (1) this battleship is enormous—as big as a football field—and (2) I am alone in a tiny rowboat trying to stop it with marbles!

Because of the confusion caused by the fog, I have the idea that if I can just throw those marbles hard enough, I will eventually pierce the hull and sink the battleship. I can even hear some of my marbles pinging off the side of the ship as I throw them, so I'm convinced that I'm causing major damage. Although I tell myself with conviction that soon I will have conquered my "little problem," it will obviously never happen as long as marbles are all I have to throw.

During my lifelong battle with the enemy in the ship, I kept looking for reinforcements. I talked with psychiatric professionals about my inability to control my periodic compulsions to act out sexually. The doctors shrugged and said they didn't really see sex as a problem. One told me that if I didn't like what I was doing, *I should stop*. I figured the doctors must not be too concerned about it or they would have taken my pleas more seriously.

I also asked for help from bishops and stake presidents. The church leaders would assure me of the Lord's love and concern, and suggest more sincere prayer, more diligent scripture reading, along with a broken heart and a contrite spirit. Apparently, I needed more repentance.

I felt the genuine empathy of these priesthood leaders and resolved to them, to myself, and to God that this time, I would prevail. I would slay my Goliath! Of course, those of us with a limited, mortal perspective all had in mind a wrestling opponent of similar size, weight and skill. By the way, one thing I also noticed was that talking with someone about my problem relieved my burden somewhat and made me more hopeful. But there was still a huge problem. Now I was sitting in my lonely, little rowboat, praying and reading my scriptures—before I once again started throwing more marbles at the battleship.

I have a friend who spent years living in emotional and mental turmoil. She had overwhelming feelings that she was unworthy of God's love, that she was a failure as a mother and wife, and that other people were better or better off than she was. At times she considered taking her own life. One day, I was struck by the thought that I knew something she didn't.

My wife and I sat down with our friend and I talked to her about depression. I explained that oftentimes, people feel debilitating unhappiness and assume that it is because of some spiritual deficiency. "If I were more spiritual (or righteous, or compassionate, or goal-oriented)," they reason, "I would be happy. If I am not happy, it must be because of some moral or spiritual shortcoming." I told her that depression was different from sadness. Sadness is an emotion that follows unwanted or troubling experiences and events in our lives. When bad things happen, sadness is the appropriate emotional response that occurs inside us. That's not what happens with depression.

Depression is the product of a broken brain. Something doesn't work quite right, and as a result, the depressed person is physically and mentally unable to feel and enjoy happiness. What's worse, the depressed person's emotional state may range from merely miserable on good days to intolerably miserable on bad days. Whatever the root cause may be—missing brain chemicals or disrupted electrical impulses or something else—depression is the result. It is not a spiritual malady. It is a physical disease of the brain.

If we break a leg, we go to the hospital and have a doctor set the bone and put the leg in a cast. We do not seek out a priesthood holder for a blessing and then head back to the armchair in the living room for more prayer and meditation and a recommitment to spiritual growth. Although a blessing may be helpful for the healing of the broken leg, we recognize that the Lord expects us to get medical help to fix our injury.

Disease in a broken brain, however, is often treated differently. For some reason we think that a broken brain can be fixed by praying and asking the Lord to heal our unhappiness. Because I suspected that my friend suffered from depression, I told her that I thought she needed to see a psychiatric specialist to consider that possibility.

My friend seemed surprised. This had never occurred to her before. I was also surprised. During all this time and throughout all her interactions with people close to her, it appears that no one before me had ever raised to her the possibility of depression. Eventually, she met with a psychiatric professional, was indeed diagnosed with depression, was prescribed the proper medication and blessedly began enjoying the happiness that can occur when a brain fires on all cylinders.

For years, my friend had been looking in the wrong direction for a solution to her problem. For years, she had been praying with ever increasing fervor for the Lord to remove the burden of her misery. The Lord did finally answer her prayers, but it was not in the way she was expecting. She assumed she would get direct intervention from God. Instead, God put a friend in her path that observed her and, drawing on his own experience with depression, was able to convince her to seek a doctor's help.

I believe that addiction—and sex addiction, in particular—is treated in a similar way by addicts and those around them. Sexual transgressions are second only to murder in seriousness. Sexual sins are a blatant violation of God's law and therefore evidence of a deficient moral character. Sin and immorality can only be overcome by the Atonement of Christ after faith and sincere repentance accompanied by a broken heart and a contrite spirit. In effect, God (through Christ) intervenes in the life of the sinner and purifies him of the sin. The sinner repents of his sins, focusing on his direct relationship with God and Christ, but also confesses his sins to a church leader. In some cases, church discipline follows. Through the miracle of the Atonement, the sinner is born again and becomes holy, without spot. But what about the *sex addict* and his sex addiction?

Like depression, addiction is, in large part, the product of a broken brain. One LDS neurosurgeon has documented the destructive physical effect that pornography has on the brain. It eventually incapacitates parts of the brain in the same way that cocaine or alcohol can destroy an addict's resistance to the compulsion to take those drugs into his body. Because of the neurological component of sex addiction, treating it as one would treat sexual transgression—as a purely spiritual malady—is ineffective.

One book that deals with the topic of overcoming sex addiction asserts that if lustful thoughts are permitted "to remain in our heads without dealing with [them] immediately, we begin physical, mental, spiritual, emotional, and neurological changes within us." Note that there are five types of change that lust can bring about inside us. I understand now that for years I was focusing on what I thought were the spiritual issues of my problem and completely ignoring the emotional, mental, physical and neurological components of addiction. I also wasn't enlisting the help of those most qualified to assist me on the "non-spiritual" end of the spectrum.

There is no question that I should have been looking to my priesthood leaders for help with spiritual issues and to advise me on spiritual matters. Emotional matters can be directly related to the spiritual ones, so they might have helped me there as well. Once we get into mental concerns, however, a priesthood leader is probably outside his expertise unless he has training in that area related to his vocation. A priesthood leader would only treat physical ailments if he were also a physician. Neurological problems are, of course, best left to the specialists. The way I was going, it was like rendering aid to the victim of a shotgun blast by applying focused pressure to just *one* of the many entry wounds while he bleeds to death out of all the rest.

Over the course of my adult life, I have spoken at different times with perhaps eleven priesthood leaders about my struggles with pornography and sexually acting out. They felt for me and expressed love and concern as I related my shame, suffering and frustration. All of these men recommended treatment of my problem with the balm of repentance and forgiveness through the Atonement. Although I embraced their counsel wholeheartedly, it just didn't seem to be enough to keep me from going back to my addiction.

But then things changed. I have now been sexually sober for long enough to know with certainty that I can stay sober for the rest of my life. Sexual sobriety has a specific meaning to me: no form of sex with self or any other person other than spouse. Period. It also means progressive victory over lust. This is by far the longest period of complete sobriety that I have enjoyed in many years, perhaps in all my adult life. Along with sobriety comes serenity and happiness. I recently told my wife that for the first time in my life, I am happy without an asterisk next to the word "happy."

To what do I attribute my sobriety? Interestingly, it did not come through a renewed and somehow greater commitment to abstinence from pornography and acting out sexually. I am no more serious about remaining sober now than I was all those other times when I vowed to myself and the Lord that I would never act out again.

There is also one other thing about which I am dead certain. My heart is no more broken and my spirit is no more contrite now than they were in the past. When I was molested as a six-year-old, my heart was broken and my spirit was contrite. When I talked to my bishop as a teenager about my desire to stop lusting and acting out sexually, my heart was broken and my spirit contrite. When I put my marriage at risk and first disclosed to my wife years ago that I thought I might have a problem with internet pornography that I couldn't seem to beat on my own, my heart was broken and my spirit contrite. When I went to meet with my bishop the next evening, my heart was broken and my spirit contrite.

Each time I met with a priesthood leader about trying to find a solution to my "problem," my heart was broken and my spirit contrite. Every time I spoke to my wife about my inability to stay away from pornography and then had to watch the pain in her face as she tried to understand, my heart was broken and my spirit contrite. Through the health crises my wife and I have endured where we have both sat in hospital beds hooked up to bags of poisonous chemicals and looked death straight in the eyes—and then did it again and again and again with our youngest child—my heart was broken and my spirit contrite. When I finally disclosed to my wife the extent of my acting out over the past several years and again placed our marriage on the brink of oblivion, I had a broken heart and a contrite spirit. I don't think my problem was that I lacked a broken heart or a contrite spirit. That pretty much describes my entire life.

So what was the difference this time around? In short, I finally came to understand that I had lost the war, and so I surrendered—not to my addiction, but to God. I gave up and turned it all over to Him. After the last disclosure to my wife, as I was suffering in desperate misery and unsure whether our family would remain together, I was struck by the clear impression that I needed to call a friend in another state to tell him what I had done and enlist his help. I followed the impression and made the call. The friend listened to me patiently and then he told me some things that changed my life.

First, he told me that he knew exactly what I was going through at that moment because he and his wife had been dealing with the same thing since a few years earlier. Second, he told me that my brain was broken, that I had an addiction. He said I needed to quit trying to beat it on my own because it couldn't be done. Third, he told me that there was hope for recovery and that all was not lost. Fourth, he told me about a 12-Step program called Sexaholics Anonymous (SA). He described it as a collection of admitted sex addicts who met together in small and not-so-small groups all over the country to support each other in their quest for sexual sobriety. He phoned me several times over the next few days, each time suggesting gently that I needed to get to an SA meeting as soon as I could. Finally, he quit suggesting and just told me unequivocally to get myself to a meeting.

I went to my first SA meeting on a Friday night. There were eleven other men in the room when I arrived. I was struck by how happy they all looked. I wondered if I was in the right place. For the next hour, I listened in awe as each of these men articulately shared his struggles with sex addiction, his hopes, his successes or his failures. It was inspiring. When my turn came to share, I was able to talk about everything: the loneliness, the shame and humiliation, the fear that I had destroyed my marriage, the pain I had inflicted on my wife, the desire to change my life, get away from the acting out, and simply live as I knew God wanted me to live.

As I spoke, the other men listened intently, many of them nodding or smiling quietly as I said things that were familiar to them from their experiences. Afterwards, I went to dinner with several of them and they explained to me how SA worked to keep people sober. I went to another meeting on Saturday morning, and another on Monday morning, and another on Tuesday evening, and another on Wednesday evening, and another on Friday evening. I have attended meetings less frequently but regularly ever since.

A remarkable thing about SA is the way it exposes addicts' secrets to the light of day in a safe way and in a safe place. One of sex addiction's biggest hooks to control the addict is secrecy. Like an infection, the shame and fear that accompany the addict's actions, thoughts and behavior remain hidden inside the addict where they fester and grow cankerous. The more miserable and isolated the addict becomes, the more he feels compelled to medicate away his misery by acting out with his drug—even knowing that the fix will only last a short time and that greater misery and isolation will follow.

When I go to SA meetings, those of us attending are able to bring all the shameful secrets out into the light. We don't speak in a salacious way, but respectfully and with reverence to the fact that the addiction is bigger and more powerful than we are. We acknowledge repeatedly during the meetings that we are powerless over our addiction, that our lives have become unmanageable, and that only God can restore us to sanity. In between meetings, we call each other on the phone.

Sometimes we call because we are having a rough day dealing with the addiction or some resentment that could give rise to a desire to act out. Sometimes we call because we want to reaffirm to someone else our intention to remain sober for another day. Sometimes we call just to check in and say hi, because the act of checking in helps us get our heads straight, reminds us how good sobriety feels, and disrupts the addiction's pattern of leading us into isolation and resentment. I have called other members in the program when I was having trouble. At other times, they have phoned me.

Once I got a call at 11:30 at night. Even though my friend didn't say he was having a bad night, I could tell. We chatted for a few minutes about nothing in particular, expressed our appreciation for each other and said goodbye. That short phone call helped him stay sober that night, and helped remind me of how grateful I was to God for finally, after so many years, so many tears and so much pain, leading me to a place where I could recover from my addiction.

I have a sponsor now. He is one of the most remarkable men I know. His faith knows no bounds. His enthusiasm never stops. His smile is infectious. His insights are always just what I need to hear. He and I share the same profession. Like me, he is a husband and a father. And he has been in the SA program and sober for almost a decade.

I also serve as a sponsor to several men who are new to the SA program. Working with them is an opportunity for me to share the experience, strength and hope that have come to me as a blessing of recovery. It is a chance for me to save lives and saves marriages. I love to see that tiny spark ignite in their sad, tired eyes where they attend their first SA meeting—when they start to hope that maybe they've found what they were searching for—maybe this is the solution to the nightmare. I smile and tell them with confidence, "This will work—if you're willing to work it!"

One of the many slogans of 12-Step programs is "One Day at a Time." I work at staying sober and in recovery one day at a time. I recognize that I am still a sex addict and that I will always be a sex addict. That is my reality. But I also realize that if I do what is necessary, I can remain in recovery, which means complete and absolute sobriety. That is what I intend to do. Sexaholics Anonymous, with God's help, inspiration and strength, will help me do that.

The picture of my addiction inside my head has changed now. I still see myself in the tiny rowboat and the battleship is still out there.

But now, the fog has dissipated so that I can see the enormous size of my enemy and know that this battle is *very* lopsided. It is *nothing* like those two wrestlers in the ring. I know that I will lose if I just sit there by myself in my rowboat with my marbles.

But now I also see a bunch of other rowboats surrounding mine—not many, but enough—and recognize my friends from SA. They have blowtorches and drills and metal-cutting saws. They tell me to stick with them and they will show me where to cut and drill and torch to slowly dismantle that battleship piece by piece. They tell me, "We know how to chop this thing up, because we've done it before ourselves." Sure enough, I can see their battleships lying in pieces in the distance. Some are neatly stacked, while others are in a bit of disarray. But it's clear that their battleships are destroyed and they are now out there helping others dismantle theirs. One of my good friends in the program recently told me with a smile, "It takes an addict to help an addict." I believe that.

Finally, what is the power source that all these cutting tools plug into so they can be used to chop up my battleship? There is no question in my mind. It is the power of a loving God who is mindful of me, my wife and my family, and who wants us to return one day into His presence. That is my hope.

2. A Letter to LDS Wives

*What every Mormon woman needs to know about
sex and pornography addiction*

DEAR WIVES:
This letter will change your life. That's a hefty promise, I know, but it will happen. Some of what I tell you will hurt. Some will challenge what you've thought for years and will require you to adjust your view of the world, your family, your marriage and your faith—but not in a bad way. At the end, you will feel that there is some hope. There is a light at the end of the tunnel.

I am writing to you with my wife of over 20 years by my side. She and I have spent hours talking about the things you're reading right now. We've prayed together. We've shed tears together. We've made discoveries together that surprised us. We've gone to marriage counseling together and found that our therapist strongly embraces what we have experienced in our recovery.

Let's get straight to the point. This is about your husband and what has been termed the "pornography habit." Some of you have been married nearly half a century; some only a few months. Some have children in the marriage while others don't. Some of you work outside the home; some are homemakers. Some of you have husbands who travel a lot for work, or who don't travel at all, or who are unemployed. But you all have some things in common: you love your husband; you know he has a problem with pornography; and this problem hurts you more than anything you've ever experienced in your life. It cuts to the very center of what it means to be a woman, a friend, a wife and a mother. Sometimes you cry yourself to sleep because of it.

You feel isolated. You can't really talk to friends about this issue. It's embarrassing. You can't talk to your mother or sisters about it for the same reason. Maybe you've tried to discuss things with your bishop or stake president, but you just don't feel comfortable talking to another man about your husband's problem and how it affects the most intimate aspects of your marriage. You may have gone to couples therapy with him. If he refused, you may have gone to therapy alone.

Through all of this, one word crowds out nearly everything else: *Why*? Why me? Why him? Why us? If he really loves me, why does he do this? If he loves the children and cares about our family, why does he continue to search this stuff out? If he knows that it's wrong, why doesn't he just stop? If he really cares about his temple covenants and our sealing together, why does he bend and break those covenants? Didn't I feel the confirming warmth of truth years ago (or recently) when I made the decision to marry him? Why, then, haven't things turned out the way I expected? Why has he promised me again and again and again that he will stop, and yet he is back at it months, or weeks or merely days later? Why does he make and then break these same promises to the bishop? If he truly believes in a loving Heavenly Father and a Savior who atoned for his sins and mine, why is this happening? Why don't I have my "happily ever after"?

The simple truth is that your husband has an addiction.[1] His brain is broken and he has lost the ability to make decisions between right and wrong when it comes to matters of sex. He doesn't stop because he *can't*.

---

[1] Some people seem fixated on making a distinction between a pornography addiction and the other, "more serious," "full-blown" sex addiction. The viewing of pornography is merely one of the conduits by which the addict acts out on his sex addiction. It is his "drug of choice." In this writing I make no distinction between pornography addiction and sex addiction because I see no meaningful difference.

You've been worried because you've heard for years that viewing pornography can lead to addiction and can drive the addict to much more serious sins. I want to be clear about this: If your husband is repeatedly looking at pornography, he is already addicted.

Most likely, he does not know he is addicted even though he is aware that what he's doing is wrong. He wants to stop. He wishes he could. He thinks he can if he just tries hard enough, just commits with enough resolve to stop. Be assured that doing what he does makes him absolutely miserable. Every time he recommits that he will never do it again, he means it. Those tears in his eyes are real. That resolve on his face is genuine.

His addiction, however, is bigger than he is, and it will beat him every time. *Every time.* Not some of the time. *Every time.* No matter how hard he tries, no matter how much you try to change his behavior, no matter how many visits to the bishop's office, it will drag him back down. *Every time.* Remember, however, that I said there are great reasons to hope. We'll get to that.

Here is something else that you need to understand: This is not your fault. You didn't cause it. He probably brought his addiction with him into the marriage. You can't cure it. Really. Try all you want, you can't cure it. You can review the computer's history and install blocking software, and he will still be an addict. You can check the credit card statements for strange and cryptic charges, and he will still be an addict. You can follow him around in your car to see where he goes after work, and he will still be an addict. You can break down in tears and spill out the anguish of your soul to him, and he will still be an addict. You can threaten to take the kids and leave him, and he will still be an addict. You can shame and embarrass him in front of friends, family or priesthood leaders, and he will still be an addict. Whatever you do, he will still be an addict.

I will go even further because you need to hear this. Your husband's addiction is not rooted in his dissatisfaction with you. You might think it is. He might think it is and even say so. You are both wrong. If you dropped 30 pounds, he would still be an addict. If you got an augmentation and liposuction and collagen injections so you looked like a porn star, he would still be an addict. If you did things in the bedroom that you really didn't want to do, thinking that maybe this way you can keep him from looking elsewhere, he would still be an addict. If you think that viewing internet pornography together or watching raunchy movies together will "enhance" your marriage or at least make him less likely to indulge in pornography on his own, you need to know that he is still an addict. Nothing you do will cure him.

One other thing. If anyone tries to tell you that your husband looks at pornography because you're not giving him what he needs, look that guy right in the eye and ask, "Won't he still be an addict no matter how much sex I give him?"

Addiction is a disease. It has no cure. You may have been told otherwise. I am asking you right now to change your thinking. I am a sex addict. I know what I'm talking about. I know this in a way that others without my addiction apparently can't know. For the rest of my life, I will always have the disease of sex addiction. So will your husband. This does not mean, however, that the disease cannot be managed and controlled. This does not mean that we cannot find peace, happiness and complete freedom from acting out. Gratefully, there is a solution.

It is important to see the disease of addiction as it really is. Believe it or not, this is part of what creates the hope you will soon begin to feel. What if your husband was a diabetic and you told him, "If you really love me, you'll stop being a diabetic"? What if you said to him, "Get over your diabetes, or I'm taking the kids and leaving"? What if you cried to your bishop, "I just don't understand why he picks his diabetes over his family"? Sounds crazy, doesn't it? You would never do that, right? Why? You wouldn't because no amount of badgering, pleading, crying or bargaining would cure your husband of his diabetes. It would always be there. Notice, however, that I am not suggesting that you ignore the diabetes. I am only saying that you can't cure it. Your husband can't cure his diabetes either. There is no cure! While he can be careful about his sugar intake, watch what he eats, get proper exercise and take insulin shots, he is monitoring and regulating—not curing—his diabetes. The disease of addiction is the same. I can't say it enough: there is no cure! There is no cure—but there is a *solution*!

One of the questions you have been struggling with for a long time is why he does so well with his resolve, sometimes going for many months, only to fall again. Why does it seem like a vicious cycle from which he can't extricate himself? The answer is that, contrary to popular notions amongst us and jokes by late night talk show hosts, having a sex addiction does not mean that your sex engine is always on and running in hyper drive. Being a sex addict does not mean you *always* want to have sex and will have it with anyone or anything including animals, houseplants and redwood lumber.

Like the ocean's tide, addiction ebbs and flow. Sometimes it's far out on the horizon; at other times you're up to your eyeballs in it. Nevertheless, like the tide, when it goes away, it always comes back. This is why your husband can seem to be doing so well at times, so well in fact that you and he and the bishop come to think that he's cured—until he "slips up" yet again. Please remember this: like the tide, the addiction always comes back. This means that if your husband ever tells you that it's no longer a problem, you can be assured that he's either kidding himself or he's lying. I know that's hard to hear, but it's the truth.

Let me suggest an analogy to help you better understand your husband's addiction. You've seen those hi-tech windmills that generate electricity. If you look closely, you realize quickly that there's more to these things than you first thought—unless you have an engineering degree, in which case you knew all this wind power stuff a long time ago. It turns out that these windmills don't simply spin in the wind and generate electricity. The windmills' blades are actually adjustable so their angles can be modified to avoid damage in heavy winds, or else opened fully in light wind to catch every bit of push from a gentle breeze. Also, the axis on which the blades spin rotates 360 degrees so it can be turned into the wind. These adjustments are important so the operator can harness the power of the wind. In addition, they are vital when repairs are necessary. If required, the operator can trim down the angle of the blades and rotate the axis out of the wind so that the blades don't spin at all. Although the wind is blowing past the windmill, no electricity is generated because the operator chooses for this to be so.

Now let's relate this to the human sex drive. In a normal person, the blades and axis of sexual urges can be adjusted. At the right times, the sex windmill can be faced into the wind with the blades open to catch the wind and spin like crazy. At other times, the windmill doesn't spin at all even though there is a breeze. Addiction changes this.

When someone has a sex addiction, the operator of the windmill loses control of the motors that adjust the blades and axis. What's worse, the windmill "adjusts" itself by always turning directly into the wind and opening the blades fully to catch all the wind. What this means for the sex addict is that when there's not much wind, there's not much of a problem. This is when he starts patting himself on the back about how strong and resolute and armored in spirituality he is. This time, he has conquered the beast! As we know, however, he really isn't cured. When the wind finally picks up, look out! The operator quickly rediscovers that he has no control of the motors, the windmill proceeds to turn into the wind, blades spinning wildly, and a "slip up" occurs. Like the return of the ocean's tide, the wind will always come back, and so there will always be "slip ups."

I don't like the term "slip up." It suggests just a little problem, a minor setback in one's progress to self-mastery. I prefer the term "acting out," which means that the addict is engaging in behavior within the scope of his addiction. For an alcoholic, this would mean consuming alcohol. For a cocaine addict, this would mean ingesting cocaine. For a sex addict, acting out means engaging in any sexual behavior, act, or conduct with anyone other than his or her spouse. This includes self sex. Also, please don't get hung up on the analogy of the windmill. It's not perfect. It's not meant to be. The same goes for the diabetes analogy. I am just trying to help you relate to the ebb-and-flow nature of addiction. There is no cure. The wind always returns. The windmill always turns into the wind. Always. Unless the addict gets himself into the solution...read on.

Returning to the windmill analogy, we need to understand what the wind is. This is another one of those things that will require you to rethink some beliefs and assumptions you've had for a long time. If I asked you what the wind might represent in relation to the sex addict's windmill, I bet you might say it was something like internet pornography, trashy movies, inappropriate television shows, and magazines that glamorize immorality. In other words, the temptations of the world create the wind. *Wrong.* The wind makers are surprisingly not what you think they are.

The wind is actually caused by debilitating negative emotions or feelings such as resentment, negativism, anxiety, fear, guilt, shame, humiliation, remorse, loneliness, anger and rage. Take a good hard look at that list again. When these emotions clog our spiritual and mental circulatory systems, they cause us spiritual, emotional, mental and even physical pain. For the addict, the way to deal with the pain is to medicate with his "drug."

Several years ago, I contracted viral meningitis. It started with a headache that proceeded to develop into a pain in my brain and spine so severe I could taste it. I ended up in the hospital with doctors and nurses coming and going with masks on their faces to avoid exposure. At first, I didn't think I needed anything for the pain. I'm one of those guys who think a little pain is a good thing—it builds character. When it grew unbearable, however, I finally accepted the morphine offered by my doctor. I think this was the only time in my life I ever had morphine. Although I did not have any addictive reaction to the drug such as an overwhelming urge for more, I did notice how the drug affected me. It didn't take the pain away completely, but it did take the edge off so that it was bearable. I still hurt. I was still uncomfortable. But now at least I wasn't writhing in pain. It made it so I could *endure* the pain.

For the addict, his "drug of choice" is like morphine, taking the edge off his emotional pain. Thus, an alcoholic drinks alcohol, a drug addict shoots up his drug, a shopaholic shops, and a compulsive eater seeks solace in food. Similarly, a sex addict medicates by acting out sexually to release chemicals in the brain that produce the pleasant, narcotic effect that accompanies sexual intimacy. Basically, the God-given feelings and emotions that should be reserved only for intimacy between husband and wife are hijacked by the addiction and used to take the edge off the perceived emotional pain through which the addict is suffering. I say "perceived emotional pain" because often the cunning addiction will fabricate painful emotions in an effort to propel the addict down the pathway to acting out and self-medication.

My addiction's favorite fabricated emotion seems to be resentment. I find myself generating resentment against other people based upon real or perceived slights, snubs, conflicts or disputes. Back before I knew anything about addiction, I would begin a downward spiral into despair and emotional pain and would eventually find myself acting out. Now that I know about my addiction and recognize its triggers, I am aware of resentment. When I feel it, I can often break it down and analyze it. Why am I feeling this resentment, I ask myself. More often than not, I find the resentment to be smoke and mirrors, of no substance at all. I recognize that it is my addiction trying to get me to give it some of the drug it craves.

For your husband in his sex addiction, it is not the pornography or the magazine or the movie that entices him. It starts in his head long before the sexual material ever hits his eyeballs. Something is going on that makes his addicted brain want to medicate. His addicted brain then goes in search of its drug. When the opportunity to view pornography presents itself, he has no defense because his addicted brain won't allow a defense, and he acts out. If no opportunity to act out appears imminent, the addicted brain becomes first anxious and then desperate, eventually fabricating the circumstances necessary to justify acting out. Fantasy and obsession are huge parts of addiction.

This is why simply resolving to avoid pornography does not work. The addicted brain goes to work to come up with reasons, situations and justifications for acting out and the addict is drawn to the drug as surely as metal shavings are drawn to a magnet. Pornography is just the drug of choice that "medicates" your husband's broken and addicted brain.

Once you understand the nature of addiction, you will understand why watching pornographic movies with him will not "help" him. Such conduct merely feeds his addiction. He goes for a ride on his addiction. Sadly, you are just there as a passenger, usually in the backseat. Submitting to things in the bedroom that you don't feel good about in an effort to be more "compatible" with your husband is also ineffective. God gave you those feelings in your heart and those thoughts in your mind for a reason; listen to them. Do not go down that path if you know it's not right. It will not make you happy. It will not save your marriage. It will not cure his addiction. You cannot fix him by sexually acting out with him.

Now, about that hope I promised you. First, you now know what you're up against. You can put a name on it. You can research it. You can read about it. You can pray about it. It is no longer confusing and unknown to you. Next, consider what else you now understand: your husband has an addiction; the addiction ebbs and flows; there is no cure; it is bigger and more powerful and more cunning than he is. What this allows you to accept is that your husband truly *does* love you, but his addiction prevents him from fully manifesting that love to you through complete fidelity to you. He *does* care about the family, but his addiction stops him from being the father he should be. His temple covenants *are*, in fact, important to him, but his addiction makes it impossible for him to keep those covenants. He wants to be worthy of the priesthood he bears, but his addiction literally puts worthiness out of reach. Where, you ask, is the hope? The hope comes in recognizing that he truly loves you and wants you at the center of his universe. The *addiction* is the enemy here, not your husband!

To add to the hope, you should also understand that while there is no cure, there is a solution *that works*! In 1974, a man who had been suffering for years from the destructive effects of sex addiction had the inspiration to attend an Alcoholics Anonymous (AA) meeting. He immediately recognized that the 12-Step program used to help alcoholics achieve sobriety could also be used to help those afflicted with other addictions, including sex addiction. He began attending AA meetings regularly and working the recovery steps with a sponsor. He achieved sexual sobriety. A few years later, Sexaholics Anonymous (SA) was born.

Members of SA meet throughout the United States in small and not-so-small groups to support each other in their efforts to achieve and maintain sexual sobriety. They meet in one-hour meetings, usually in the evening, during which they share their experience, strength and hope with each other. These meetings are life changing. At these meetings, the sex addict finds that he is not alone, that others suffer as he does, and that many of them have found the sobriety that has eluded him. The new member quickly finds a sponsor, another person further along in recovery, who acts as a mentor to help the new member achieve and maintain sobriety. In addition to attending meetings, the SA members call each other to check in, to offer support, or to ask for help.

Let me help you understand what is going on here and why it works. First, addiction thrives on loneliness, shame and despair. This is one reason why addiction is so difficult to overcome. The more entrenched the disease becomes, the more isolated and guilt-ridden the addict becomes. It is a downward spiral. Second, the one thing that addiction hates is the light of day. If you think about the times when you have talked with someone about your husband's problem, you may have noticed that the act of disclosing to another person lifted a weight from your mind and heart, even if only for a short time.

It is the same with addiction and SA. If the addict can talk about the addiction with someone else who knows and understands exactly what he is going through, the power of the addiction dissipates. His resolve to stay sober increases. His desires to act out lose their compulsive power. He begins to address those negative emotions that are at the root of his emotional pain.

Some people have the notion that these meetings are full of sickos looking to swap stories and share the secrets of the trade. To the contrary, these meetings are full of people who sincerely want to change their behavior with God's help and then to help others change their behavior as well. They tend to be well-educated, religious, family-oriented, and friendly. Newcomers often express surprise at the optimistic atmosphere of the meetings. This keeps them coming back.

It is important to know that SA may be the only program out there with the ability to help sex addicts find a *lasting* sobriety and a solution to their problem. It may be that nothing else works! That is not hyperbole. In my experience, it is fact. Psychiatric professionals acknowledge that the program is effective. Members of the clergy who counsel parishioners on matters of addiction acknowledge this as well. Recovering addicts themselves acknowledge this. It works!

In addition, there is a support program for you, the wife, called S-Anon and it is available to you whether your husband attends SA or not. Its mission is to help relatives and friends of sex addicts find support and comfort. Again, newcomers are surprised by the friendliness and warmth found in these meetings. The relief that comes from finding others with similar circumstances and experiences is palpable. My wife enthusiastically invites you to join her and the other women of S-Anon. Share their experience, strength and hope! Your husband needs SA now! You need S-Anon now! His life, your personal sanity, your marriage and your eternity together may very well depend on it. Please find meetings and begin attending. Do whatever it takes to get there. Please understand that this is not merely one of several equal and interchangeable options; in our experience, it is the only option!

Sexaholics Anonymous advocates a definition of sexual sobriety that is easy to understand. Sexual sobriety means no form of sex with self or any other person other than one's spouse. It also means progressive victory over lust. It is a clear standard, and if you think about it, it is the Gospel standard.

After trying and failing countless times over the years to achieve sobriety on my own, I began attending SA meetings and working the steps. I have now been sober long enough to know that I can stay completely sober for the rest of my life. That means no acting out—ever. That means no more "slip ups," no more "mistakes," no more "giving in to temptation." I know a number of SA members (many of them LDS) who have achieved significant years of complete sobriety. I know that this solution and the program work! Until I began attending meetings and working the steps, I had trouble stringing together even two weeks of sobriety. Meetings in SA have saved my life! One thing that is so important to me is that I can look my wife in the eye, tell her that I am sober, and have her know exactly what I mean.

I realize that one of the biggest tools that addiction has in its bag of tricks is denial. Men will not stop the car to ask for directions because they deny ever being lost. Similarly, men will not admit to sex addiction because their denial mechanism keeps telling them that they can take care of this thing on their own—they just need a little more prayer, a little more time, a little more will power, and this thing will be licked! Remember the parable of the ocean's tide: the addiction always comes back! He will never beat it *on his own*. Give him a copy of this letter and ask him to read it. I wish I could promise that it will solve all your problems, but I can't. Addicts are a difficult bunch to convince, especially about their own addiction. Find a copy of my essay "Sitting in a Rowboat Throwing Marbles at a Battleship" and have him read it. Give copies of both essays to your bishop and your stake president. Ask them to talk with your husband.

When I finally disclosed to my wife the nature and extent of my sexually acting out, she was devastated. She wanted to die. She was fortunate, however, to have a close friend who survived similar circumstances a few years before and had found recovery through S-Anon. In tears of despair, my wife cried that she just wanted someone to tell her that there was some hope. With quiet confidence, her friend told her that there most definitely was hope, that we could both recover together, and that our marriage and love for each other could achieve a strength, confidence and unity beyond anything we had known before. I lack words to express how right she was.

Please don't give up hope.

3. The ABCs of Porn Addiction

The real reasons why so many LDS men can't kick the pornography problem

I BRIEFLY CONSIDERED calling this "The Essay No One Wants to Read," but then decided to plunge in and call it what it is, an explanation of exactly what keeps so many Mormon men from being able to find a permanent, bullet-proof way of staying away from pornography and compulsive sexual behavior. Before I do so, however, I want to make three points as background. First, although my intended audience is primarily Latter-day Saints, I am not suggesting that Mormons are any worse off in terms of pornography and sex addiction than society in general. We're not. Many, if not most, men in America these days have significant problems with pornography and compulsive sexual behavior. For a fair number of these men, the response is simply to shrug and not to worry about it. "Men will be men. That's how we're wired. Gotta satisfy the urges or it'll make us 'unhealthy.'"

In contrast, I think that a large percentage of our Mormon men are suffering so badly right now because they are unable to live a life of integrity and are miserable as a result. They repeatedly and inexplicably engage in sexual behavior they know to be wrong and it is eating them up on the inside. In addition, a significant number of our women are struggling and suffering because they are unwilling to buy into the false but commonly-peddled notion that women just have to accept that "their men will be men"—pornography and masturbation are just part of the package. For Mormons—and others—something in our hearts and minds is telling us that this just isn't the way it's supposed to be. This isn't what God intended.

Back From the Abyss

Second, I speak from the position of one who has been to hell and lived to tell about it. I am a recovering sex and pornography addict. For years, I acted out secretly on my addiction. During those same years, I fought to overcome my "little problem" like a man possessed. I refused to let it suck the life out of my marriage and my family. I refused to let it steal my soul. Until I found real recovery, however, my addiction was entirely indifferent to the depth of my devotion to faith and family, and methodically sucked and stole away at its leisure. That's what addiction does.

Finding Recovery

Third, when I talk about being an addict in recovery, the emphasis is on *recovery*. Being in recovery means that I used to act out on my addiction but now I don't—at all—ever. This doesn't mean I'm somehow "cured" and will never have to worry about compulsive sexual behavior ever again. Like a recovering alcoholic, I will return to my drug if I ever quit working my program of recovery. The exciting thing for me, however, is that I've finally found a recovery path that works. It has enabled me to stop engaging in the behavior that was killing me and killing my marriage.

Before recovery, my wife and I both felt like we were sliding off separate cliffs into oblivion and just barely holding on by our bloody fingernails. Then one day, I stopped. I surrendered, gave it all up, turned it over to a loving Father in Heaven who had been patiently waiting for me, and walked away from it. Again, this doesn't mean I just started to ignore the problem and miraculously it went way. I walked away from the addictive behavior by walking into a program of recovery that included therapy and 12-Step meetings.

I can now look my wife straight in the eye and tell her I'm sexually sober. I couldn't do that before recovery. She knows my sobriety date and knows how long I've been sober. She knows that with God's strength and blessing, I have repented and forsaken the sin. She looks back into my eyes with confidence, knowing that finally I have the ability to stay sober and never go back. Before recovery, she wasn't able to do that. Things are much different now. I am able to live a life of integrity. My wife is able to live a life without fear.

Along with others in recovery, I have found what countless Mormon men are dying to find but failing: complete sexual sobriety. My wife has found what so many Mormon women would give up everything to have: a sexually sober husband. We don't say this lightly or by way of boasting. We are talking about it because we want other people to have what we have—or simply to know that it is even possible.

We want to see LDS husbands and wives with confidence in each other. We want to see Latter-day Saint women who trust their husbands, who don't cry themselves to sleep at night, who don't wonder what happened to their "happily ever after." We want to see Mormon men worthy of the priesthood they bear, worthy to lay their hands on their children's heads and utter blessings that are too wonderful to describe, worthy to attend the temple with their wives and feel the presence of angels, worthy to stand as disciples of Christ having felt the full redemptive power of His Atonement. We want to see our people enjoying peace and love in this life with no secrets gnawing away at their insides.

The purpose of this essay is not to talk so much about how my wife and I found recovery from my addiction or what we do to stay in recovery. That story is told in detail on our website at *RowboatAndMarbles.org*. Instead, as noted above, I am focusing here on why so many Mormon men are failing to find lasting recovery from sex addiction and why some of them seem incapable of truly forsaking the sins of pornography consumption and extramarital sexual behavior including masturbation. The goal is not merely to shake a finger and pontificate about what's gone wrong. Rather, we want to discuss why the things we all keep trying—whether as addict, spouse, or priesthood leader—don't work and will never work—because they *can't* work. We need more people in the Church to understand the reality of the "pornography problem" and then go to work with the tools that can actually help men and women overcome our generation's greatest challenge.

The Addiction Recovery Relationship

Pornography and sexual addiction can be described by way of a simple relationship: $a => b$, $b => c$. We call this the Addiction Recovery Relationship. It's really that simple: "a causes b, and then b causes c." This relationship, properly understood, will allow priesthood leaders, parents, spouses and addicts to see what must *always* happen in order for an addict to find and stay in recovery.

The three elements of the Addiction Recovery Relationship are (*a*) debilitating negative emotions, (*b*) lust, and (*c*) sexually acting out. Of the three elements, c is the one that Latter-day Saints focus on most. It represents what some men (and women) do to act out sexually: the viewing of pornography, masturbation and other compulsive sexual behavior including serial affairs, fornication and acting out with prostitutes or anonymous partners, to name only a few possibilities. Latter-day Saints know that this behavior is wrong. We receive counsel from the pulpit to avoid all such conduct, whatever the cost. We teach our children to stay away from it. We put filters on our computers. We try to avoid immoral television programming and magazines. We exercise selectivity in the movies we see. We might even picket adult establishments to run them out of town. We expend an enormous amount of energy fighting to get *c* out of our homes and lives.

For addicts and those around them, however, there is a problem. Usually, we addicts do all the stuff that we *think* is required of us. We either confess to the wife or parents or else they catch us. We then confess to the bishop—sometimes. For the millionth time, we jump back into prayer and scripture study with renewed zeal. We take our repentance very seriously this time (just as we did the other 999,999 times we tried to stop). We go to great lengths to eliminate from our lives all of this *c*. Before long, however, it's back again just like the ocean's tide. Whenever we go to battle to get rid of *c*, *b* just generates more *c*. It's always going to be like that unless we do something to deal with *b*.

Lust is the Real Culprit

As I said above, *b* is lust. It is the thing we are actually addicted to. My definition of lust is when we wrongly and selfishly use ourselves, other people or things in an attempt to satisfy our own appetites regardless of consequences to ourselves or others. This is much more complicated than the idea that lust is when a man thinks dirty thoughts about a woman. It is also apparent that my definition of lust involves more than just sex. Although lust could concern food, money or power, I am going to focus on lust primarily in the context of sex.

Lust is what motivates the addict. When lust rears its ugly head and roars, the addict runs off to find something to feed it. Lust doesn't really care so much what it eats just as long as it gets fed. Very often, the food most readily available for lust is pornography and masturbation. To get what it wants, the disease of lust addiction strangles the parts of the addict's brain that constitute his conscience, the parts that normally keep him on the straight and narrow and away from sin and immorality. As I said above, lust is like the ocean's tide—it ebbs and flows. Except in extreme cases, lust is not a 24-hour-a-day obsession. Depending on many factors, it may at times be just a tiny blip on the radar while at other times it may crowd out everything else. Sometimes it doesn't bother us at all; later, it overwhelms us.

Addicted to More Than Just Porn

In the Church, we refer frequently to a "pornography addiction." This is a misnomer. The pornography addict is actually addicted to lust. His "drug of choice" happens to be pornography. In discussions of alcoholism, I've never heard anyone refer to a Belgian beer addict, or a Mexican tequila addict, or a Russian vodka addict, or a peppermint Schnapps addict. A person addicted to alcohol is addicted to alcohol *in all its forms*. Similarly, a person addicted to lust is addicted to lust *in all its forms*, not just pornography.

If a man is addicted to lust with his "drug of choice" being pornography, and he then swears off pornography, he is still addicted to lust (the *b* in our Addiction Recovery Relationship). All he is doing at this point is merely abstaining from one discrete aspect of *c*. Since he is addicted to lust (*b*) in all its forms, it is very unlikely that his exclusive means of self-medicating is by viewing pornography only. The lust addict acts out with pornography, masturbation or *anything else* that will give him the lust hit his addiction demands. In other words, if a guy has a "pornography problem," you can be assured that *pornography is not his only problem.*

Returning to my point, if a lust addict commits to stop consuming pornography, it is similar to an alcoholic committing not to drink beer. That commitment is only meaningful if the alcoholic understands that he must also abstain from the consumption of *all* alcohol, not just beer. To achieve recovery from lust addiction, the addict must commit to abstain from lust in *all its forms*, not just pornography.

I have heard of men who have admitted to their wives that they view pornography from time to time, but who have assured them that it never goes so far as masturbation. Often it is the wife who repeats this assertion, partly because of a lack of understanding, partly because of denial, and partly because of a co-addictive desire to somehow shield or protect her addict husband from the full consequences of his behavior.

In any event, this is always a head-scratcher for me. First of all, pornography and masturbation are like conjoined twins. If one walks through the door, the other can't be far behind. Second and more importantly, talking about the viewing of pornography without any accompanying masturbation as though it were somehow a positive thing is akin to saying that an alcoholic only drinks vodka but fortunately doesn't mix any tequila in with it. Alcohol is alcohol. Lust is lust.

Even if it's true that our hypothetical friend "only" looks at pornography, he is still doing nothing other than feeding the "starving" lust monster inside him. If he masturbates, he is feeding the same monster. If he reads racy spy novels with graphic sex scenes, he is feeding the same monster. If he goes to R-rated or NC17-rated movies loaded with nudity, sexuality, vulgarity and immorality, he is feeding the same monster.

Whether he looks at the Sports Illustrated swimsuit issue, or Playboy, or some other "adult" magazine, he is feeding the same lust monster. Whether he goes to the mall to stare or goes to the beach to leer or goes to a strip club to do more than just look, he is feeding the same lust monster. Saying that someone *only* looks at porn occasionally but doesn't masturbate is hardly reassuring when both activities feed the exact same lust addiction inside the addict.

Fantasy, Relationship and Connection Addictions

We are all pretty accustomed to pointing fingers at lust in the forms that are most familiar to us. Internet pornography, raunchy television shows, vulgar movies and smutty magazines are easy targets. Once we understand that lust is the true enemy here, however, we quickly make some other realizations that are going to rock a lot of boats out there.

Let's take me as an example. It turns out that I'm not just a pornography and sex addict. I am also a fantasy addict, a relationship addict and a connection addict. All of these are behaviors that I acquired as a child and then perfected as an adult. They were my coping mechanism.

When I was a child, I disappeared into a fantasy world where the women accepted me, liked me and were happy to see me. When my reality hurt me, I went to my non-reality fantasy world where I hurt less. After I was exposed to pornography and sexual abuse, the fantasy women took on the appearance of the women in the magazines. As a child, lust became my anesthetic. Even when I went for years without looking at any pornography, my fantasy world was populated with enough pornographic memories that it was for me almost no different than looking at the "real thing."

Now Connecting

My relationship addiction and connection addiction go back to my early years. I had a mentally ill mother whose mental illness, it turns out, stemmed in large part from growing up in the home of a sex addict. Today, I describe my childhood as life with an alcoholic—only without the alcohol. Coming home from school each day was riddled with anxiety because I never knew which version of my mother was waiting for me. Because of that emotional instability at home, I developed a compulsion to connect with other women. As I said, I longed for someone who accepted me, liked me and was happy to see me. I was constantly looking for a girl or a woman I could connect with—not necessarily in a sexual way, but in some elusive mental-emotional-spiritual way.

Much of my young life consisted of trying to make connections with women in whatever ways I could think of. A compliment from a female teacher sent me into orbit. An appreciative laugh at my humor from a girl in a high school class would keep me medicated for the rest of the day. A smile from the lady at the cash register at Safeway made me feel euphoric. Eye contact with a woman in an elevator or in the car next to me in traffic energized me for hours.

I would do whatever I could to make a connection somehow, never realizing that that's what I was doing. If a connection wasn't possible or practical, I would fantasize about making the connection. *What could I have said to make that woman back there interested in me? How would she have responded if I had said this or that? What would I have said then?* I would fantasize over the missed connections and the almost-connections. I had no real consciousness of what I was doing, but doing it made me hurt less.

In reality, I was addicted to lust and what I was doing was feeding my addiction. Each of those attempts at making a connection was a "lust hit." Whenever I drifted into fantasy, I was inhaling lust. When I was self-medicating on connections, pornography didn't have to be anywhere in sight for me to feed lust. It also turns out that pornography, and internet pornography in particular, was an extension of my connection addiction. Each new image was a hopeless attempt to connect somehow with the object of my lust. For me, women had lost their identity as women and daughters of God, and had become instead objects for me to use in my never-ending quest for that last great connection that would bring peace and harmony to my universe. I had no concern for what they thought or how they felt, and cared only about how they could make me feel. I only cared about the connection.

The Facebook Nightmare

This idea of a connection addiction is important for Mormons as we try to understand what works to help those who are now suffering in silence and genuinely don't understand why they keep getting crushed and dragged under again by their "little problem." Similar to consuming pornography, looking for connections is a way of feeding lust. What this means is that internet flirting is feeding the lust monster. Facebook, in my opinion, is a wide-open opportunity for lust-addicted men and women to indulge in fantasy, connections and relationships, with each interaction providing one more hit of lust. Facebook is a nightmare for lust addicts.

Lust Without Sex

With this new understanding of the different faces of lust, we can now take a fresh look at the man who leers at women in public places (whether real or virtual) and maybe has a tendency to comment on their appearance and physical characteristics. We know he is feeding his lust. If such a guy shrugs, chuckles and says it's harmless and he isn't doing anything wrong, we know better and we can clearly articulate what he is doing and why it's a huge problem.

What this also means is that some men find ways to act out and feed their compulsive desire for lust through conduct that is apparently non-sexual. Men who show inordinate physical affection or who constantly seek interaction with women other than their own wives may knowingly or unknowingly be feeding a lust addiction.

To those who would protest, I respond, "Hey, if I'm wrong, then prove it. With the obvious exception of your wife, cut off all your interaction with women—other than the bare minimum required for work and household tasks such as shopping. Do that for two weeks." If there's no addiction, such a man won't miss a thing. If, however, he finds himself bouncing off the walls, restless, distracted and irritable, maybe he should consider this lust and connection addiction model we've been talking about here. Maybe he's feeding his lust and maybe he's doing it entirely without pornography.

Floating Off Into Fantasy

A fantasy addict is obviously someone who compulsively floats off into mental fantasy as a way of self-medicating. Fantasy can often be sexual but doesn't have to be. Regardless, the fantasy produces lust hits for the addict and allows him to "act in" on his disease rather than act out. While he may be completely abstinent from pornography, his addiction to fantasy is causing pretty much the same effect on his brain as if he were sitting in front of a computer monitor or holding a magazine. The same lust addiction is being fueled, pornography or not.

No, It's Not Innocent

A relationship addict is someone who feeds his lust by compulsively cultivating relationships with persons other than his spouse. Once again, these relationships can be non-sexual. Friends at work, old high school girlfriends, and even the wife's friends can all be sources of lust hits for the addict. Wives often have trouble articulating that gut feeling that something just isn't right when they become aware of a relationship between their husband and another woman. Oftentimes the husband responds critically, accusing his wife of being "paranoid" or "selfishly territorial."

Indeed, some men will even go to great lengths to be transparent with these relationships in order to show their wives that there is nothing sexual and therefore nothing "inappropriate" going on. "She's a single mom. I'm just helping her out." The point everyone is missing is that a lust-addicted man—or a woman—can and will take lust hits from such a relationship even if nothing sexual is occurring, even if to the outside observer there is no evidence of anything *untoward*.

When the "friend" smiles, or waves, or calls, or texts, or goes to lunch with him, or helps him shop for his wife's birthday present, or tells him how lucky his wife is to have him, or tells him how she hopes to find a guy just like him, the relationship addict is taking giant lust hits, just inhaling as fast and as hard as he can. All the while, he is patting himself on the back for maintaining a proper, professional distance. Just because he can't be sued for sexual harassment, however, doesn't mean he hasn't poured buckets of lust down the gullet of his addiction.

Debilitating Emotions: Way Bigger Than Pornography

With lust addiction actually being comprised of fantasy addiction, relationship addiction, connection addiction, as well as addiction to pornography and compulsive sexual behavior such as masturbation, we see that we have our work cut out for us. This is *way* bigger than just pornography. We have to get at b if we ever expect to overcome c.

The problem again, of course, is that if we only focus on b, a will just continue to generate more b. Recall that the a in the Addiction Recovery Relationship is debilitating negative emotions. They include fear, anger, resentment, shame, humiliation, depression, negativism, anxiety, guilt, remorse, loneliness, and rage. While this is not a complete list, it is sufficient to make a point about what is crushing many Mormon men. Like men everywhere, they are dealing with the stresses of daily life, the finances, work issues, church callings, the children, the wife, and the marriage relationship. Most Mormon men don't drink, don't smoke, don't gamble, and don't do drugs—all substances and behaviors often abused by addicts as a means of escaping reality and anesthetizing emotional pain.

Self-medicating with Sex

One behavior that most married Mormon men (and others, obviously) do engage in, however, is sex. The sexual act causes a chemical release in the brain that makes everything feel A-OK. It is like an opiate. Sex makes people hurt less—like morphine, or marijuana, or alcohol. Like actual drugs, sex can easily be abused in order to give an individual a hit of pain relief. When an individual wrongly and selfishly uses himself, others or things in a sexual way to feed his own appetites (i.e., to self-medicate so he hurts less) regardless of consequences for himself or others, he is feeding lust and he is or is becoming addicted to his drug just the same as if he were acting out with cocaine. Like all humans, Mormon men (and women) are susceptible to using sex to feed lust and to self-medicate.

The Real Cost of Objectification

I want to say a few words about objectification. Objectification means viewing another human being and seeing only the physical characteristics while denying or ignoring that there is any soul, mind, heart, thoughts, needs, desires, emotions, concerns or anything else that might identify the object as a human being and a child of God. *Every* person who compulsively views pornography necessarily engages in objectification. As addicts, we have to divorce the object of our lust on the computer screen from any notion that it is a son or daughter of God and created in His image. If we did not do so, the fantasy of the experience would die immediately and our addiction would not get its lust hit.

Whenever I hear a man say that looking at an attractive woman is like enjoying a beautiful sunset, or like gazing at a priceless work of art in the Louvre, I say, "You have proven my point. You don't see that woman as a daughter of God. You see her as an object without a soul. She is something less than how you see yourself, something less than human. To you, she is merely paint on a canvas that serves nothing more than to tantalize your senses—or, more accurately, your lust. You see that woman as eye candy. That, my friend, is objectification, and that, my friend, is at the core of lust addiction." You cannot look at pornography without objectifying the individual you are looking at!

Although what I have just described is pernicious enough, objectification does not stop when the computer switches off or when the magazine is closed and hidden away. As a component of lust addiction, objectification progresses and intensifies just as the addiction does. In *all* cases, men who view pornography begin to view the actual women around them as objects. In their minds, they strip away the soul and humanity until only the body is left, and then they fantasize about the body.

Despite those men who will swear up and down that I'm crazy and that they are the exceptions because they have some magical, unknown and unknowable immunity to this particular component of lust, I will go on record to state that objectification can and *does* extend to one's wife. Men who look at pornography necessarily objectify their wives. The wife becomes just another object to be used for the husband's sexual gratification along with all the other objects of fantasy in the addict's lust-compromised mind.

If a husband then commits to quit the porn (again focusing on nothing more than a tiny sliver of *c*), his addiction to lust (*b*) most likely continues unabated. Why wouldn't it? He continues to objectify the women around him, including his wife. He uses her selfishly to feed his appetites without regard to the consequences to her.

For those who would dismiss pornography as harmless or at least harmless to all but the one who looks at it, I point to the collision of objectification and the wife. Heavenly Father has given women a wonderful gift of being able to connect physically, emotionally and spiritually with their husbands. Connection with her husband on all these levels is one of the most important aspects of a married LDS woman's existence, just as it is for the married LDS man. Men who view pornography, engage in masturbation or otherwise indulge in lust, however, cannot bond emotionally or spiritually with their wife. When that sacred bond is disrupted by the husband's secret, "victimless" behavior, the wife feels it in her heart and knows it in her mind. She may not be able to attach a name to the objectification, but she is most definitely aware of it. She knows something isn't right in the marriage.

If an LDS woman unknowingly marries a pornography and sex addict, she will soon feel a sense of loss, a hole in the marriage where emotional and spiritual strength and support were supposed to be. Once an LDS woman discovers that her husband has been feeding his lust by the viewing of pornography and masturbation, and has also included her in his sex routine—not as his eternal companion, but as an object to stimulate and satiate his lust—the effect is devastating to her on every level: physically, mentally, emotionally and spiritually. Every time he acts out, whether she is aware of the act out event or not, she experiences the subsequent carnage and it wounds her mind and spirit as an exploding grenade would wound her body. The pain that comes from finally realizing what role she plays in her husband's sexual acting out is searing. Therefore, a husband who indulges in pornography and any extramarital behavior including masturbation can only do so by having no regard for the well-being of his wife.

Why Mormon Men Can't Kick Their "Little Problem"

With all the components of the Addiction Recovery Relationship on the table now, I'm prepared to state why so many Mormon men can't kick the pornography problem. Although it's probably obvious at this point, here it is: If a pornography, sex and lust addict is not actively seeking treatment for *a, b, and c*—for all three elements of the Addiction Recovery Relationship—he will never get into permanent recovery. If he does not deal with *a*, it will always create more *b*; if he does not deal with *b*, it will always result in more *c*.

If we think that all we have to do is give a guy a calendar and tell him to put an X on the days when he doesn't look at porn, we are dreaming. If we think that simply putting the computer in a high traffic area in the home will guarantee no more acting out, we are *still* dreaming. If we think that starting each day with prayer and scripture study will *by itself* wash away the years of mental, spiritual, emotional and physical damage caused by porn and masturbation binging, we are keeping ourselves blissfully ignorant of the bedlam addiction leaves in its wake. If we think that a wife can "cure" her husband with Sunday night check-ins and little chats about how the efforts to "fight temptation" are going, we drastically underestimate the monster we are fighting. If our recovery plan does not squarely address the crushing problems of lust addiction and debilitating negative emotions that we have been discussing, we will continue to fail.

Men are contemplating suicide nowadays because none of the flimsy suggestions for "fighting temptation" work for lust addiction—they can't possibly work because they don't treat *b* or *a*! For these men, their acting out progresses to where they feel they've reached a point of no return. Death begins to look preferable to more of the misery and painful downward spiral into insanity. If the proposed treatment of the "pornography problem" (or whatever you want to call it) does not address *a, b, and c*, there will be no recovery! Too many Mormons are focused on slapping little Band-Aids on *c* behavior without any consideration whatsoever for the physical, mental, emotional and spiritual chaos going on in the areas of *b* and *a*.

"But…But I Really Just Have a 'Little Problem'!"

One of the objections addicts will have to what I'm saying is that all this *clearly* has nothing to do with them; they just have a "little problem" that occasionally involves pornography (but *never* masturbation, of course). Such men couldn't possibly have any kind of lust addiction because they say their prayers, read their scriptures, do their home teaching, bear their testimonies on fast Sundays, love their wives and children, are diligent in their callings and are altogether *far too spiritual* to be addicted. They don't fit the stereotype—whatever that is. Their reasoning, however, is defective.

Mormon men do not return again and again to pornography and compulsive sexual behavior unless something is compelling them to do so. *There is only one thing that repeatedly compels undesirable sexual behavior and that is an addiction to lust.* The reason men act out on lust is because they are trying to numb debilitating emotional pain. Whether they are aware of the underlying trauma or not and whether they admit it or not, it is there. If there were no pain, they wouldn't be trying to self-medicate to cover it. If a man keeps going back to pornography after repeatedly trying to stop, it is because he is addicted to lust. Lust is compulsively attractive because it numbs emotional pain. This is why addicts are addicted. When dealing with pornography and compulsive sexual behavior, there is no such thing as a "little problem."

The Glorious Banner of "Accepting Personal Responsibility"

I've talked about a lot of difficult things. If a pornography and sex addict were to read this, his mind would be reeling right now. For many reasons, he believes his very survival depends upon identifying arguments about why what I'm saying here doesn't apply to him. Because he just has a "little problem," the banner he will wave most furiously will be the glorious banner of "accepting personal responsibility." It all flows from how addiction impairs the addict's ability to think. It makes it so he often can't recognize reality and, even if he can, he doesn't care about reality because his compulsions, when they are fired up, don't allow him to care about anything but feeding the addiction.

The Relativity of the Addict's Reality

This is one of the huge problems associated with addiction that is wiping out men both inside and outside the Church. But it is a very complicated issue. Like I said, addicts often can't recognize reality. One of the ways this manifests itself in the addict is when he takes actual truth and warps it to create an artificial reality that fortifies his addictive world.

A good example of this was Elder Ballard's talk in the October 2010 General Conference in which he talked about addiction. Although he spoke specifically about prescription medication abuse, he made it clear that the principles applied across the board to all addictions. While the talk was dead-on and helped in furthering understanding of addiction in the Church, something happened near the end that was significant. Elder Ballard said that if an addict wants to get over the addiction, "[i]t begins with prayer—sincere, fervent and constant communication with the Creator of our spirits and bodies—our Heavenly Father." While he was right—recovery can and often does begin with prayer—I thought as I was listening that two things were going on in the minds of addicts in the Church as they also listened to him at that moment. (When I talk about addicts here, I mean addicts who are not in recovery from their addiction. They are either currently acting out on their addiction or merely doing essentially nothing to find and effectively achieve recovery.)

"Lord, Can I Get Over This Problem on My Own?...Um, Never Mind."

When Elder Ballard uttered that simple phrase, "It begins with prayer," every addict listening to the message unconsciously added two little words. What they all heard was "It begins *and ends* with prayer." Their broken brains tweaked the message enough to continue to justify—at least in their own minds—what they had been trying and failing to do for years: overcome addiction in isolation by means of prayer and willpower. Like I said, Elder Ballard was accurate when he said it all *can* begin with prayer. If an addict would employ sufficient humility and willingness to offer a simple prayer, "Heavenly Father, can I get over this problem on my own, or do I need help from other people?," the Lord would respond with clarity, "Get help." The problem is that addicts *never* ask that question. There are reasons for this that I'll get to in a second.

The other thing that many addicts were doing as they listened to Elder Ballard was frantically making a list of as many reasons as they could about why Elder Ballard's message on addiction applied to someone other than them. Until I got into recovery, I didn't see myself as an addict. Like so many other men in the Church, I genuinely believed that I just had a "little problem," not an addiction. Eventually, after my behavior progressed and grew more compulsive and when even my broken brain could no longer say that I just had a "little problem," I was finally compelled to adjust my defective thinking so that now I believed that I was evil, slothful and destined for hell—but I still didn't think I had an addiction.

The word "addiction" carries with it a host of connotations, one of which is "out of control," which in turn carries with it the suggestion of insanity. No one wants to admit to insanity for several reasons. Three of the biggest reasons—at least for addicts—are fear, shame and humiliation. The fear leads them to say, "If I am insane, I will lose my job and the ability to provide for my family. I will also lose my wife and I will lose my children because they will not want to stay with an insane person—especially an insane person who is addicted to pornography and compulsive sexual behavior. Finally, the nature of my conduct will cause me to lose my membership in the Church."

For most married men in the Church, the only three things that truly matter to them are their wife, their children, and their membership in the Church. If they were to admit to addiction, they believe that what would inevitably follow would be the loss of all three. They would be left with none of the sources of joy in their life and instead would have only the source of continuing misery—their addiction. This is why addicts never ask the Lord that question about whether they need help from other people. They don't want to face a possible reality where they are addicted to sex, unemployed, insane, divorced, estranged from their children, and excommunicated. Instead, they are desperately screaming on the inside, "I can fix this—*on my own!*"

Three Short Sentences

Three short sentences are killing Mormon men: "This is my problem to deal with. I created this mess, so it's up to me to clean it up. Nobody else has to get involved." As far as addiction is concerned, I don't think the problem is that Mormon men are refusing to accept personal responsibility. Quite the opposite, I believe nearly every man in the Church who currently suffers in silence with his sex and pornography addiction is hiding behind the notion that because he needs to be a man about it and accept personal responsibility, he needs to (or gets to) take care of it on his own.

The principal of personal responsibility has been hijacked by addicts as a justification for remaining in isolation. The fact that so few men in the Church regularly attend 12-Step meetings to assist their recovery from addiction is evidence that pretty much everyone in the Church with the "little problem" is desperately holding out for the Lord to make this all go away as a reward for this demonstration (in isolation) of their acceptance of personal responsibility. For addicts, "accepting personal responsibility" is really just cover for what their addiction craves: isolation. "Accepting personal responsibility" nearly killed me. It has killed other men.

Summing It Up

We've talked about the many reasons why a large number of Mormon men are unable to kick the "pornography problem." Pornography is just one sliver in the wood pile of acting out options for those addicted to lust. When we focus exclusively on abstaining from pornography, we will *always* fail because our addiction to lust will merely compel us to act out in other ways. If we wait long enough, the lust addiction will even eventually drive us to act out with pornography again. Lust addiction is not just addiction to pornography, but is also made up of connection addictions, relationship addictions and fantasy addictions.

Without recovery, we addicts can fuel lust indefinitely even with no pornography in sight. Men who lust necessarily objectify women and this objectification extends even to their own wives. Debilitating negative emotions create emotional pain which pushes the addict to self-medicate with his drug of choice. He feeds lust because lust makes him hurt less. Sex and pornography addicts inside and outside the Church are doing whatever they can to continue conning themselves and others that all this addiction stuff has nothing to do with them; they just have a "little problem." And speaking of the "little problem," LDS men gladly accept full personal responsibility for it—because doing so allows them to continue to fight their losing battle on their own, in isolation.

Calendars with little Xs on the porn-free days are not going to solve this complex and monumental problem. Keeping our days occupied with "positive and uplifting activities" won't either. Singing a hymn or reciting a scripture won't do much if anything to address the depression, rage, resentment or fear that is compelling the addict to self-medicate. None of these tiny Band-Aids, by themselves, will even begin to cover the gaping, gushing wounds of lust, connection, relationship and fantasy addictions brought on by debilitating negative emotions.

"It Seems So Hopeless!"

Not long ago, my wife was talking to a friend about our view of the pornography addiction problem in the Church. The friend shook her head despairingly and said, "How can you stand to look at it in this way? It seems so depressing! It seems so hopeless!" We don't see it that way at all.

Thousands of years ago, the children of Israel stood crowded and cornered on the banks of the Red Sea. The armies of Pharaoh were bearing down on them. Annihilation seemed inevitable. The situation was hopeless. Then Moses turned to face the flood and raised his arms.

From somewhere in the eternities, the God of Abraham, Isaac and Jacob invoked His omnipotent will and the waters of the Red Sea parted to the left and to the right. The children of Israel passed over on dry land and the waters then came crashing down into their place again, destroying Pharaoh's armies.

For years now, hundreds of thousands if not millions of Mormon men have—along other men worldwide—been struggling to overcome pornography addiction and compulsive sexual behavior. Rather than our men getting stronger, however, it appears that the compulsions are the ones getting stronger. We are losing the battles; we are losing the war. The casualties—husbands, wives, children, families, and communities—have been immense. As individual addicts each in his own isolation, we have proven definitively that we cannot overcome this enemy by flying solo. The situation is indeed hopeless. But...

When we addicts, along with our parents, spouses and priesthood leaders, finally come to see that we have lost the war, individual miracles will take place. Like the children of Israel, when we finally see the utter futility of our predicament, we will turn to God—for real this time. We will each say, "Heavenly Father, I am beaten. I can't do this anymore. It is hopeless! I need You to do for me what I can't do for myself. I need You to change me where I have been unable to change myself. In the past, I told You what I was willing to do to 'repent.' I told You how I was willing to go *just this far*—and no further—to overcome my 'little problem.' I told You that I expected this to be sufficient. I am different now. Before, I was willing to give away half my kingdom to know You. Now, I am willing to give up *all of it*. I am willing to do *whatever it takes* to get well, to beat this addiction, to find sexual sobriety, to achieve recovery. *Whatever it takes.*"

The Men Among Us

There are men among us who have found true sexual sobriety. They are addicts in recovery. In the past, they obsessively viewed pornography and engaged in compulsive sexual behavior. They no longer do so. They have completely stopped. After years of failure and futility, they have finally forsaken the compulsive behavior and that in turn has enabled them truly to repent of the sin. They have been to hell and lived to tell about it. As they became willing to do whatever it took, and then actually did whatever it took, Heavenly Father changed them on the inside. They reacquired their integrity. They now have a message and the message is this: Recovery is possible and it is wonderful!

Find these men. Ask them what is necessary to get into recovery. They will smile and then they will tell you just what you need to do. They will also promise you, "This will work if you're willing to work it." They will talk to you about therapy and 12-Step meetings and getting a sponsor and working the 12 Steps. They will teach you how to identify all of the lust triggers in your life and how to eliminate them. They will teach you what it means when someone says, "I finally came to realize that as an addict, I am entirely unable to 'lust like a gentleman.' I am allergic to lust in all its forms." They will help you recognize and accept that you truly are powerless over this addiction and that only Heavenly Father has the power to overcome it for you.

You will be momentarily disappointed because you will have been hoping for a magic bullet, a kind of spiritual inoculation that only stings for a second but then guarantees that you will never be tempted by lust again. Such a shortcut happily is not on the menu. Heavenly Father requires that we each do this *the right way*.

Despite the disappointment, you will remember that prayer uttered on the shores of your personal Red Sea with the armies of Pharaoh (lust) about to crush you. You will recall your moment of hopelessness when you turned to the Lord and said, "I am now willing to do whatever it takes. *Whatever it takes*." These men will show you what it takes.

If Moses Had Other Plans

Something to keep in mind about the children of Israel is that when God parted the sea to the left and to the right, they still had to walk right down the middle on the path the Lord provided. It wouldn't have worked very well if Moses had said, "I think I'll wander down the beach a ways and see if I can't find my own way across. No hurry. I'm a pretty smart guy. I'm feeling pretty strong. I'm feeling pretty confident. I'll get this figured out at some point—on my own."

Recovery is attainable right now. Many of us have found it and we are ready to share it. In fact, we are required to share it. The only way we can hold onto it is to give it away. To those who say, "It sounds so hopeless," I reply, "Absolutely! Isn't it great! The only thing we can do now is to *turn to God and live*. I was one of the hopeless ones. Now I'm not. Heavenly Father saved me from the destruction of addiction. He changed me when I couldn't change myself. It is my experience, strength and hope that with God, nothing is impossible."

4. Porn Addiction is Like a Muck Fire in My Brain

Why merely stopping the porn binging isn't enough

IN FLORIDA, FIRE DEPARTMENTS have to deal with an unusual type of blaze called a muck fire. Muck is dirt that contains a lot of decomposing plant material and is usually found under lakes or swamps. Occasionally, when the water table goes down, the muck can dry out. As the chemical process of decomposition progresses, muck generates heat. Finally, when lightning strikes or someone carelessly tosses a cigarette out the window on the highway, the muck can ignite.

Muck fires pose a serious complication for firefighters. Unlike regular forest fires, a muck fire burns underground. It can't be seen, although it can be smelled. The firefighters try to control above-ground forest fires by building fire breaks. They have to be vigilant to control the fire. If they see a hotspot getting ready to cross the break, they focus their equipment on that area to prevent the fire from jumping. The problem with muck fires is that because they travel underground, they can pass right below the firefighters and the fire breaks and spring up on the other side to start another blaze above ground.

A muck fire can burn for months, even years. It smolders quietly, often without anyone being aware of it. When dry weather creates the right circumstances, the muck fire pops out of hiding and starts another forest fire. Once firefighters locate a muck fire, they need to till the soil to churn up the embers and get them out in the open where they can be extinguished. Because of its makeup, however, some muck can even be resistant to water. It is a difficult problem to handle. If firefighters aren't vigilant or leave too soon, they can later discover that the fire really wasn't extinguished; it just went underground.

A muck fire is a lot like fantasy in the mind of a sex addict who is trying to control his behavior and avoid acting out on his addiction. Like a firefighter, the addict thinks he can watch vigilantly to make sure the fire of his addiction stays in a controlled burn mode. If temptations to act out arise, he tries to douse them or smother them. Eventually the fire of compulsion and desire subsides and the addict breathes a sigh of relief because he thinks he has won another round in the battle with his addiction. Through vigilance and firm resolve, the addict comes to believe that he has taken control of the fire. Little does he suspect that his addiction has muck fires of its own. And just like the muck fires, it turns out that his addiction has merely gone underground.

My first exposure to pornography came at age six. An older boy in my neighborhood showed a magazine to me as a means of grooming me so he could molest me. My next exposure came at age eleven when I found a magazine as I was emptying the kitchen garbage in a dumpster down the row from our townhouse. I hid it in the bushes in my backyard. I went back to look at it a couple times, but since I knew it was wrong, I took it and threw it back in the dumpster. When I couldn't get the images out of my mind, however, I eventually returned to the dumpster, fished out the magazine and hid it in my backyard again. At some point, the magazine lost its allure and then I threw it away for good.

I was thirteen when two friends and I found a magazine in the orchard behind our homes. Some other kid had hidden the magazine in the old stacked fruit bins we used to climb around in. We looked at it together and then went our separate ways for the day. I returned later in the evening and moved the magazine to another location so no one else could take it.

I was again exposed to pornography at ages sixteen, seventeen and eighteen. Later, during my two-year mission for the LDS church in a European country, I frequently had to avert my eyes as I walked down the sidewalk to keep from gazing at the pornographic poster ads pasted on what seemed like every bit of outside wall space in the city. Newspaper stands also presented a problem with the covers of raunchy magazines hanging right at eye level when I walked by.

Once I realized what my eyeballs had latched onto, I fought the compulsion to look twice. Usually I prevailed and was rewarded with a feeling of satisfaction, as though I were bigger and stronger than the smut, and so imbued with God's power that I could not fail to win the battle if not the entire war. How naïve I was. Satan must have had a lot of good laughs as he watched me in my earnestness, fighting the good fight. Satan could afford to be patient. He understood muck fires. I didn't.

During graduate school, I got my first internet connection and within months had discovered a strange and horrifying new world. What had before required going to a video store or a convenience store was now available in my home—for free. I started binging. My grades suffered. My wife suffered. My sanity suffered. My addiction was patient in its methodical conquest of my will and brain. Still, I fought it. I battled with the ferocity of a man desperate to save his marriage, his family, his career, his financial future, and his soul. Tears, vows to quit for good (I really mean it this time—as if this time will somehow be different from the ten thousand other times I vowed to quit!), confessions to wife and bishop, heart-felt professions of faith in the infinite power of the Atonement of Jesus Christ.

I left every General Priesthood Meeting for 25 years inspired and more resolved than ever that I would never allow myself to fall back into that hellish cesspool of misery again. I would stay away for a while, sometimes for years, but like a yo-yo, I always went back. As I said, I stopped ten thousand times. "Stopping wasn't my problem; staying stopped was."[1]

I am grateful to a loving Father who answers prayers. When finally

---

[1] I wasn't the first person to say this, but it certainly describes my situation perfectly.

I cried, "Lord, if thou wilt, thou canst make me clean," He responded, "I will." Thirty-five years after that first image flipped a switch in my brain, God sent an angel to save me. He came in the form of a long-time friend from back in my mission and college days. Rather than appearing in a flash of heavenly light, he simply spoke with me on the phone. I will never forget his peculiar choice of words. From his own experience, he said, "My friend, your brain is broken." Wow. It turns out I didn't lack resolve or sincerity or faith or contrition or humility or a noble pre-earth lineage. My brain was broken, plain and simple. I had an addiction; I was addicted to sex. I couldn't get over it on my own.

Despite all my solemn affirmations that the Lord was on my side, I later came to learn that getting over this "problem" on my own (i.e., without the Lord) was exactly what I had been trying to do for decades. I was setting up the framework of what I was willing to do and then demanding that the Lord and my addiction comply *with my terms*. It's as if I had been praying and saying, "Please, Lord, take this burden away from me! I will do whatever it takes—as long as it doesn't involve anything more than praying really, really hard with my eyes all squinched up to show how serious I am—oh, and as long as I don't have to tell anyone!" Effectively, I was saying, "Take this burden away from me, Lord, because I'm not willing to do whatever it takes on my part to get rid of it."

My friend helped me connect with Sexaholics Anonymous and I have been attending two or three meetings a week ever since. I have a sponsor and frequently talk with him and others on the phone or after meetings. I have been working through the twelve steps based on the recovery program of Alcoholics Anonymous. When I finished the seventh step, my sponsor told me I could now raise my hand in meetings to identify myself as willing and available to sponsor newcomers. I cried.

Sexaholics Anonymous helped me get completely sober for the first time in decades. It saved my life. When I talk about sexual sobriety, I mean nothing more or less than "no form of sex with self or any person other than husband or wife." Not much ambiguity there. I also mean "progressive victory over lust." I have been completely sober for long enough now to know that I can remain completely sober for the rest of my life. Like Job, I have experienced "things [that were] too wonderful for me to know." I can now look at my wife, tell her I'm sober, and see love, trust and happiness in her eyes. It feels wonderful. I told her in a quiet moment a while back, "This is where I always wanted to be."

In these recent months, I've learned a lot about myself and my disease. Much of it I hadn't wanted to know in the past. Happily, it appears that I now possess sufficient humility and clarity of mind to see that my continued recovery depends on accepting that there is no cure for the disease of sex addiction and that it is a progressive and degenerative disease. This means that it is not going to go away, and that, without treatment, it will get worse with time until it kills me. Giving me great hope, however, is the knowledge that the solution I've found in Sexaholics Anonymous stops the progression of the disease and helps me sidestep its effects. This means that I do not presently act out on my disease, and that as long as I work the program of recovery and stay in the solution, I will never act out again. This doesn't mean, however, that I'm cured; it just means that I've found a solution to the problem that works.

Not long ago, my view of sex addiction was turned on its ear. As I said, I used to think that I was winning the war. Those gaps of several months or even years between bouts of binging on pornography both as a child and as an adult were, to my mind, progressive victories. The way I saw things, I had successfully fought off the adversary for years with only an occasional "slip up."

For a long time, I figured that the internet connection was what ultimately did me in. Until then, I thought I had things under control—more or less. After all, the Lord was on my side. I assumed that the internet with its easy access to pornography was what led me to become an addict. I thought I had turned the forbidden corner some time in my thirties and it was only then that my "little problem" became a full-blown sex addiction that nearly killed me. I was wrong about this. It turns out I had been an addict since the age of six.

There was a missing link in my understanding of addiction, and that link was fantasy. In my view, fantasy is the part of addiction to which most people, addicts especially, fail to give proper deference. This applies not just to sex addiction, but to every other addiction out there as well. Alcohol, cocaine, shopping, gambling, eating, sex—it doesn't matter; fantasy is a component of the addiction. It is not a by-product of addiction; it is the very mortar that cements together the cinderblocks of addiction until they become the seemingly insurmountable walls that surround, isolate and imprison the addict. Because fantasy is a component of addiction, it does no good to counsel an addict that the simplest and most effective way to overcome the addiction is just not to think about it. *Thinking about it is the addiction!*

Consider this: You can't just tell alcoholics to quit thinking about alcohol and expect that this simple advice will somehow cure them. If it were really that easy, there wouldn't be any alcoholics. They would all just quit thinking about alcohol, and BAM! problem solved. It turns out that our brains are a little more complex than that. Addiction, too, is more complicated than that. Addiction to a particular substance is not just about the substance. It also involves what the brain is doing prior to the body's consumption of the substance, during the consumption, and after the consumption of the substance.

Have you ever heard of a "dry drunk"? "Dry drunk" is a term used frequently in Alcoholics Anonymous, often by the members in reference to themselves. A dry drunk is an alcoholic who, although sober and not drinking in the technical sense, is drinking inside his head by means of fantasy. A dry drunk's thinking becomes muddled and impaired in much the same way that an actual drunk's brain would be muddled and impaired.

The reason for this is that when the brain begins to think about its drug of choice such as alcohol, it starts secreting pleasure chemicals in anticipation of the arrival of the drug. If the drug never arrives, the brain has to content itself with the self-produced chemicals. They aren't the drug of choice, but for the addicted brain, they are better than nothing *and* they have the effect of increasing the mental pressure on the addict to go find some of the "real" drug. A dry drunk can put himself into a drunken stupor by fantasy alone. Usually, he doesn't know he's doing this. In fact, he's probably patting himself on the back about what a good job he's doing at keeping sober. Not surprisingly, a dry drunk has a much greater chance of becoming a wet drunk than a person who is actually sober.

The classic image is that of the alcoholic sitting alone at the kitchen table. In front of him on the table is a bottle of whiskey. He sits staring at the bottle. His mouth is watering. Sweat drips off his brow. Nevertheless, he is resolute. With determination, even defiance, he growls that he is stronger than the bottle and that he's not going to give in. He sits there for hours just staring and sweating. Finally his will prevails over the bottle (or so he thinks), and he stands up and walks out of the room.

Those ignorant of the complexity of addiction might view this as a point in the win column for the alcoholic. In reality, it is a loss. Addiction: 1; addict: 0. If you had looked closely at this guy at the kitchen table, you would have noticed his hands. They were gripping the sides of the chair so tightly that his knuckles were turning white. If an alcoholic is "white knuckling," he is already drunk, even if the bottle never touches his lips. He is drinking in his head. He is feeling the burn as the whiskey rolls down the back of his throat. He is feeling its warmth expanding slowly out of his stomach into his extremities. He is feeling the effects of the alcohol as it numbs the pain and sweeps away the cares, worries and inhibitions in his head. Like a muck fire, fantasy is raging in his mind while he sits stolidly at the kitchen table giving no outward indication of the inner turmoil—other than the white knuckles. In effect, he has consumed his drug without even touching it.

Why doesn't he just stand up, walk out of the room and quit thinking about it, you ask. Good question, but only because it illustrates a misunderstanding about addiction. Because of the hook of fantasy, walking away from the drug doesn't make the addictive compulsion subside. In fact, the addict *can't* walk away from it because his muck fires are in his brain, not in the bottle. Remember that I talked earlier about how addiction involves more than just the drug. Fantasy is the missing link. Fantasy is a major component of addiction. The image of the man at his kitchen table staring at the bottle is only a metaphor. He may be walking his dog in the park, or stuck in traffic, or on an elevator, or singing hymns in church. The bottle of liquor doesn't even need to exist. All the addict has to do is conjure up the image of the bottle in his mind—either deliberately or accidentally, it doesn't matter—and the addiction goes to work from that point on.

Once you put fantasy into the sex addiction equation, you can see why it is so pernicious. It is much more than merely "thinking dirty thoughts." Unlike pornography, fantasy is a flighty target. Fantasy doesn't exist outside of us. It is the product of our own minds. We have a hard time dealing with the issue of fantasy because we really don't like to revile and point fingers at ourselves. To hate the purveyors of fantasy is to hate ourselves. After all, we are responsible for it!

What's more, fantasy keeps the addiction front and center even if the actual drug is a million miles away. This is why fantasy is so much like a muck fire. If we got rid of all the pornography on the planet, sex addiction would still be alive and well and resting quite comfortably in the form of fantasy in the minds of addicts. It can smolder and keep the fire burning in the addict's head for years. While he may be sexually sober in the technical sense because he doesn't look at pornography and he doesn't act out with other people or himself, his mind still provides fertile ground for the muck fires of fantasy, smoldering and very much alive. Sex addicts can be "dry drunks" just like alcoholics. And very few people seem to understand this. Until recently, I certainly didn't.

For years, I thought the ultimate enemy was pornography. I could quantify my perceived success in the war by counting the months or years since my last pornography binge. By my way of seeing things, more time since the last binge meant greater strength, greater success, and greater spirituality. See, this time around, I had really meant it when I vowed that it would never happen again!

In reality, I was using the wrong unit of measurement. Pornography was my standard, when in fact *lust* was the more accurate unit to measure my sex addiction. If I had charted out my "success" based on the pornography standard, the graph would have looked like a mountain range with peaks, plateaus and valleys representing longer periods of abstinence, interspersed with much shorter periods of binging. If I had used the *lust* standard, however, it would have looked like a tidal wave growing progressively larger as time went on. I wasn't winning at all. Quite the opposite, it was a massacre. Addiction: 5,232,017; addict: 0. I was a "dry drunk."

In the reality we live in, lust is a slippery thing. By contrast, pornography is easy: all pornography is bad, therefore any pornography is bad. If pornography comes around, we know to flee, to get ourselves out, just like Joseph in Egypt, fleeing Pothiphar's wife. Lust isn't as simple. When lust rears its ugly head, we can't flee it, because it is inside us. Since we can't run away from it, we actually have to deal with it. From what I've been told by apparent non-addicts (assuming they are telling the truth), when lust arises, they just change the channel in their head and think of something else. For "regular folks," that may do the trick. For addicts, unfortunately, it just doesn't work that way.

I smile sadly when I hear someone suggest that singing a hymn or reciting a scripture is a good way to "replace inappropriate thoughts." Nope. At least not for the addict. "Inappropriate thoughts" hijack the addict's mind and become nothing less than obsessions. Singing a hymn or reciting a scripture is like sitting in a rowboat throwing marbles at a battleship. They make a delightful ping when they bounce off the hull, but the battleship is still coming straight at you and is going to smash you to bits.

When a skunk crawls under your front porch and dies, you don't start hanging up air fresheners and hope no one notices the smell. You roll up your sleeves and go to work. You tear up the front steps, put on a mask and rubber gloves, and drag the bloated carcass into a double-lined plastic bag so you can haul it off. You can sing a hymn or recite a scripture if you want, but you still have to do the dirty work to get rid of the stink.

For me, getting rid of the stink has involved months of counseling and therapy to deal with the stuff in my head that was compelling me to self-medicate. As part of my 12-Step recovery, I am making lists of each resentment I've felt and every wrong I've ever done. It has been painful, it has been hard, and at times it has been embarrassing. But it has also been absolutely necessary.

The sources of the bad smell in my life include being molested as a child, being emotionally abused in my childhood and adolescence, and suffering a lifetime of depression. I spent 35 years trying to bury my hurt, shame and humiliation only to discover that, like zombies, they kept digging themselves out and showing up on my doorstep. And they smelled much worse than dead skunks! Since coming into recovery, I have been tilling the soil of the graveyard in my mind to make sure all the zombies are rooted out and aren't going to pop up later at inopportune times. Whether muck fires or zombies, it can sometimes be rotten work. Still, it beats the alternative, which is more of the addiction and more acting out and more misery.

One thing I know is that addiction thrives on secrecy. The more secrets I hold onto, the more resentful and isolated I feel, and the more likely I am to act out with my "drug of choice." By bringing the secrets out into the light of day, I eliminate the cancerous places inside me where addiction can fester. As I have "dried out" and become sober, I have been able to experience life with all its ups and downs, its good and bad, without the constant need to self-medicate. Fantasy has lost its hook. Its shiny allure is gone because I now see it for what it is. Like Dorothy, I've pulled back the curtain and found that the mighty Oz—the fantasy in my head—is nothing more than a strange miserable little man—my addiction—pulling levers, flipping switches and twisting knobs, all in an effort to keep me believing that Oz is real.

So as not to be misunderstood, I am not making light of addiction or fantasy when I reference *The Wizard of Oz*. They are not be trifled with. They will kill me if I don't take them seriously. I am also not suggesting that merely reading about addiction and fantasy will cause a light bulb to go off in the reader's mind and suddenly all his problems will be solved. To the contrary, recovery from addiction is hard work. It is progressive but slow. It requires the help of other people. To put it another way, you can't recover on your own! In my opinion and based on my experience, Sexaholics Anonymous is a necessary component of my continuing recovery.

I am no longer a drunk—dry, wet or otherwise. I am living proof that there is hope for those who continue to suffer from sex addiction in shame and silence. No more muck fires. Sobriety and recovery are attainable and they are fabulous!

5. Another Letter to the Wife Who Suffers in Silence

*How LDS women can know if their husbands are sexually sober—
and what to do if they're not*

[The following is a response to an internet forum post by an LDS woman who was trying to make sense of things after discovering her husband's pornography and sex addiction.]

TO THE WIFE Who Suffers in Silence:
I'm the guy who writes the rowboat and marbles essays about recovery from sex and pornography addiction (*RowboatAndMarbles.org*). I've been in recovery (i.e., no porn, no masturbation and progressive victory over lust) for long enough now to know that complete and lasting sexual sobriety is possible both for me and for other LDS men. Although I've seen a number of LDS men find this same recovery, sadly I've seen many more that don't. I have come to recognize some trends.

First, those who get into and stay in recovery do four things: complete honesty with their wife or some other person, complete honesty with their bishop, therapy with a professional person experienced in treating sexual addictions, and active participation in an effective 12-Step group more than two times a week. Second, those who don't get sober and find true recovery don't do those four things. This is not to say that this is absolutely the only way to get sexually sober and stay in true recovery. I don't know that it is. What I do know, however, is what I've seen and what I've seen is that men who stay in recovery do those four things while those who fail to recover don't do them.

Most of the LDS men I see who fail to stay sober tend to view therapy and 12-Step as unnecessary inconveniences for men of their intelligence, strength and spirituality. They think these things are crutches for the weak among us (apparently, that would include me). Those of us in actual recovery scratch our heads. We're indeed weak and yet we're completely sober sexually. They're strong (at least in their own minds) but can't seem to string together more than a couple weeks without porn and masturbation. In recovery, we're happy and getting happier. They, on the other hand, continue to be scared, confused and miserable.

You said your husband has gone to support groups but they haven't helped. It's important to know that not all support groups are equally effective. This is certainly true with 12-Step groups. The Church's pornography addiction support group (PASG) unfortunately tends to be in the fledgling stages in many areas where it exists. These meetings often lack the experience, strength and hope of men who have achieved long-term sobriety and who can help lead the newer men in the program to sobriety. Without men in serious recovery, these meetings can end up being a group of scared, embarrassed, ashamed and humiliated men who sit and talk about how sorry they are and how much they love Jesus. This is not an effective 12-Step meeting. Also, the Church's 12-Step groups tend not to have sponsors, another key component of effective 12-Step groups and recovery.

Oftentimes, LDS men will attend twelve meetings of the Church's PASG program (one meeting a week for three months, one meeting for each of the 12 Steps) after which they announce to their wife and their bishop that they've been miraculously cured of their "little problem." Probably, they actually believe this, as do the wife and the bishop. They're not cured, however, as they will find out again a few weeks or months later when they once again find themselves acting out and lying about it.

In contrast, many LDS men are finding sobriety in 12-Step groups outside the Church. In particular, Sexaholics Anonymous (SA) is very effective. It is my experience and that of many others that SA is the best way for LDS men to deal effectively with pornography and sexual addiction. It's amazing and inspiring to see them transform from scared, ashamed, empty shells of men into the confident, worthy priesthood holders they've always wanted to be. I expect that at some point, enough LDS men will take their SA experience and sobriety with them to the Church's PASG groups and fortify them so they become effective as well.

We all need to understand that porn consumption is really just a manifestation of an addiction to lust; lust is a drug that addicts use to self-medicate with when they feel overwhelming negative emotions like resentment, humiliation, fear and anger. If a guy keeps focusing on fighting the "temptation" to look at porn, but never does anything to deal with the lust addiction or the emotions fueling the desire to medicate, he can *never* get into recovery.

Again, if a guy says he's all fixed—no more porn urges for him—and yet he can't articulate how he is treating and monitoring the lust addiction and the debilitating emotions, we know he's dreaming or lying. We have to treat the emotional turmoil, the lust addiction and the compulsions to act out sexually—all three—if we want to recover. It appears your husband isn't doing this.

So many LDS men aren't getting sober because they are trying to do it on their own in isolation—or else confiding only in people who have no experience in dealing with sexual addiction. If your husband will get an LDS sponsor who has walked the road to recovery, the sponsor will look him in the eye and tell him:

- I know what you need to do to get sober because I've done it.
- I know when you're lying because I've lied about the same things.
- I know how you think you're smarter than everyone else just as I used to think I was smarter than everyone else, too. That's how all addicts are.
- I know how you objectify the women around you just as I used to do.
- You can't fool me because I *was* who you are. I *know* you.

- I know what the overwhelming compulsion to act out sexually feels like and I know what to do to make it stop—forever.
- I can show you what to do and it'll work for you, too, if you're willing to work it.

I am one of those guys. I can look your husband in the eye and tell him what sobriety feels like and what it takes to get it. Those of us in recovery are out there and looking to share the message of hope. In fact, it is our experience that in order to keep what we have, we have to give it away to others.

You mentioned that your husband always takes full responsibility for his conduct. I've done some writing about the myth of "accepting personal responsibility" and urge you to read it in "The ABCs of Addiction." It turns out that "accepting personal responsibility" is a hallmark of LDS men who want to be left alone so they can isolate with their addiction. They've conned themselves and those around them into believing that because they're "manning up," they're taking this seriously—and this time it'll work—if only everyone will just leave them alone. Their addiction admires and appreciates these men immensely when they "man up"—it means more time acting out and more of the drug it craves.

I think you're absolutely right to ask yourself the questions you ask and to feel the emotions you're feeling. When wives ponder their future with their addicted husband, it is vital that they protect themselves—physically, mentally, emotionally and spiritually—from their husband's behavior. One way they can protect themselves is to understand reality. This is reality: A man cannot get into recovery and stay there simply by prayer, scripture study and willpower.

Like diabetes, addiction requires treatment and monitoring. That treatment includes therapy and one or more 12-Step programs. Any man who is not following an active recovery program specific to sexual addiction but who is telling his wife that he no longer has any compulsion to act out sexually is unduly optimistic or simply lying—or both. Addicts who aren't in recovery are liars. It's part of being an addict.

Many women wonder how they can know whether their husbands are in true recovery. The answer lies in listening to spiritual inspiration, responding to gut feelings and keeping in mind a simple riddle from Alcoholics Anonymous:

Question: What is the difference between an addict and an addict *in recovery?*

Answer: You can't get the addict to talk about his recovery and you can't get the addict *in recovery* to shut up about it.

If your husband is in recovery, he will attend 12-Step meetings, he will read the literature, he will get a sponsor and work the 12 Steps with him, and eventually he will become a sponsor and help other men get sober. Most importantly, if he is in recovery he will spontaneously share with you new experiences and insights of sobriety as he progresses in recovery.

If he is not sharing spontaneously it is because he has nothing to share. If he has nothing to share, he is not in recovery. There are only two possible camps in the sex addiction recovery world. Either the addict is actively working toward recovery through a defined program and will stay sober, or he is not working toward recovery and is basically blowing in the wind. This second guy is either acting out currently or merely treading water until the compulsions once again overwhelm him and he slips up as he always has.

As you said, you can't work your husband's recovery for him. He has to do that. One thing you don't have to do, however, is pretend along with him that he is getting better when he's not. Everything you've described about your husband indicates that he's *not* in recovery and never has been. Sure, he's been penitent at times. Sure, he's desired to change at times. But he's never been in recovery. You can tell him that. Because you know he's never been truly sober, you can tell him that all your decisions from now on will be based upon the fact that he is not in recovery.

You can also tell him that other LDS husbands are achieving complete sexual sobriety now and that you deserve nothing less than that. Now means *now*, not three months from now, or six months from now, or a year from now. By the way, in case he wonders, complete sexual sobriety means no pornography and no masturbation—ever. It also means progressive victory over lust. Recovery does not mean trying really hard and only slipping up once every three to six months. We have another name for that: active addiction.

I mean it: You are a daughter of the God of this Universe and you deserve nothing less than a sexually sober husband. Ask him if he is willing to do whatever it takes. He owes that much to you and he has the ability to give you what he owes—if he is willing to do whatever it takes. If your husband wants to talk about what it takes, he can e-mail me.

If you feel like talking with an LDS woman who has achieved recovery from her husband's sexual addiction, I know several of them who would be happy to visit with you by phone or e-mail. They will give you a strong plug for attending S-Anon meetings, a safe and inspiring place where LDS women are finding strength and healing from the trauma caused by their husband's behavior.

As you know, no one can guarantee that your husband will get sober and stay sober. What these women will help you do, however, is learn how to recover from the bombs your husband has been dropping on you for your entire marriage and even before that.

God bless you and every woman currently suffering as you are. We're praying for you. Don't give up hope.

6. Getting on the Same Page

12 changes Mormons should make right now to their thinking about pornography addiction

LATTER-DAY SAINTS can make a difference in the struggle against sex and pornography addiction, a battle raging for the souls of God's children. One big problem we have, however, is a hand-wringing, stomach-churning fear that we have no idea what we're talking about. The following points can help get us all going in the same direction against a cunning enemy that we must understand and see as it really is.

1. We Need to Quit Speaking in the Future Tense

"If you don't stop looking at pornography, you are going to become addicted." We need to quit talking about what's going to happen—because it has already happened! We should say this instead: "You are unable to stop looking at pornography because you are addicted." Addiction loves denial. In fact, it depends on it. The longer the addict stays in denial, the longer the addiction gets its drug.

When well-meaning people around the addict keep encouraging him to stop the "little problem" before it turns into the big A-word(!), they are unwittingly abetting him in his denial. When an addict hears the future tense, his addicted brain rejoices and he says to himself, "See, there's still a chance for me to fix this thing by myself. I just need more resolve, more determination, more faith and more time—*on my own!*" He couldn't quit the last time—or the time before that or the time before that or the time before that—because he was—and remains—addicted. Let's get ourselves into the present tense. He is not going to become anything *because he already is*!

2. We Need to Quit Calling It a Pornography Addiction

We should call it a sex addiction. Although this will shock a lot of folks, I'm not trying to be controversial. Like I said, I'm just trying to get people to see the enemy as it really is. Actually, it's not even really a sex addiction. It's more of a lust and fantasy addiction. Addicts disappear into lust and fantasy as a means of self-medicating and escaping a painful reality. Sex addicts feed their compulsion for lust and fantasy by acting out with their drug of choice, often pornography because it is so readily available and can be consumed in secret.

When we call it a pornography addiction, we minimize the scope of the crisis and again facilitate the addict in his denial. There were periods of time in my life when I didn't look at pornography for years. Because I couldn't see that I was a lust and fantasy addict (most addicts can't), I thought I was beating my "little problem" and winning the war. I wasn't. Lust and fantasy were destroying me. The type of addiction we're dealing with here lives on in the addict's brain even when no pornography is present. Take a look at the essay "Porn Addiction is Like a Muck Fire in My Brain."

Think about alcoholism for a minute. Why don't we say, "That guy has a 'Coors Light in 12-ounce cans with the lid popped and served very chilled' addiction"? Sounds nuts, doesn't it? Why? Because we recognize that the problem is not cold Coors Light. We wouldn't even say our friend has a *beer* addiction. The alcoholic is allergic to alcohol *in all its forms*. It's the same with pornography. Pornography is the Coors Light of sex addiction. It is just the vehicle by which the sex addict brings *lust* and *fantasy* through his eyeballs and into his brain.

I'm not suggesting that we ignore the fight on pornography. I believe quite the opposite. But I'm also saying that we need to understand that the enemy here is much larger in scale than just pornography. The true enemy is addiction to lust and fantasy. All pornography addicts are addicted to lust and fantasy and are therefore sex addicts. If we put filters on the family computer and move it to a high-traffic area, we minimize access to pornography, but don't really get at the real culprits that are snuffing out lives and destroying marriages: lust and fantasy. This is so much more than a pornography addiction for everyone involved.

3. We Need to Understand that "Repentance from Sin" and "Recovery from Addiction" Are Not the Same Thing

They are interconnected, but they are not identical. Addiction is not sin; repentance is not recovery. Sex addiction compels a person to sin, but it is not the same thing as sin. Likewise, just because a man repents of his sins, it does not automatically mean that he has entered recovery from his sex addiction. This explains the baffling plight of the addict who has repented so many times he can't count them anymore. Why does he keep going back to the pornography and compulsive sexual behavior? Is it because his repentance isn't sincere enough? Does he not cry hard enough? Does he not have enough resolve or conviction? Is his heart not broken? Is his spirit not contrite? Or is it maybe something else?

Is it possible that the issue is not a lack of *repentance from sin*, but rather a lack of *recovery from addiction*? If the addict does not get into true recovery from his addiction, his addiction will continue to pop up days, months, or even years later, at which point the compulsions will once again overwhelm him, and he will once again act out—even though he was completely sincere in his repentance and absolutely firm in his resolve to forsake the sin.

Addiction has spiritual, emotional, mental, physical and neurological components. For this reason, recovery from addiction requires more than "traditional" repentance from sin. The compulsive viewing of pornography and acting out sexually in other ways are manifestations of an addiction to sexual lust. Sexual lust is "an inordinate thought or feeling that drives us to use ourselves, others, or things for self-centered destructive purposes." It is a broken brain's attempt to numb its pain through self-medication.

The source of the pain is debilitating emotions or feelings such as resentment, negativism, anxiety, fear, guilt, shame, remorse, loneliness, anger and rage. Unless an addict can get into recovery and deal with them, these runaway emotions will continue to cause pain, the addict's brain will continue to feel the compulsion to medicate with lust, and the addict will end up acting out with pornography or in some other way.

If it sounds complicated, that's because it is. It is not a "little problem." This is what addiction is all about. When a guy with a "porn problem" scoffs and says he's really not "that bad off," we need to help him understand that he really is "that bad off." If he wasn't, he would have given up the pornography years ago. He can't give it up because he is addicted to it. To beat it, he needs to couple his repentance with recovery. Only then will he finally be able to forsake the sin and become free. Only then will he truly come to feel and understand the peace of God's forgiveness and the purifying effect of Christ's Atonement.

4. If We Know We're Not Qualified to Help Someone Overcome an Addiction to Lust and Fantasy, Let's Let a Professional Do It

We are all mostly well-meaning and we love to give advice. When you bring up the "pornography problem," everyone has an opinion. If, however, you mention addiction to lust and fantasy, just watch the room go silent. No one really knows what to say.

If someone is addicted to lust and fantasy, suggesting the singing of hymns and the reciting of scriptures will not solve the problem. In contrast, professional therapists and counselors who have experience in treating sex addiction can help an addict understand what is going on, why he acts out as he does, and how he can stop. Becoming a participating member of a 12-Step group will also help the addict get real support for a real addiction. We should not facilitate his denial by offering puny solutions to a monolithic—and fatal—disease.

5. We Should Accept that Sex Addiction Really Is a Disease

There's a disconnect in a lot of the thinking out there when it comes to sex addiction. People believe that there truly can be an overwhelming, compulsive power of addiction when it comes to alcohol, cocaine, heroin and cigarettes. These drugs are all tangible things. We can put our hands on them and take them into our bodies. For some reason, however, people are having trouble wrapping their heads around the idea that an addictive compulsion to engage in sexual behavior is practically identical to an addiction to the consumption of tangible drugs.

I see people nod in agreement about the addictive nature of pornography, and then the next words out of their mouths are expressions of dismay that a particular man doesn't just stop looking at pornography if he knows that it's killing his marriage. That's the point! He doesn't stop because he can't stop. He can't stop because he's addicted. Addiction means that his brain can't resist the compulsion to act out with his drug. If you think that it doesn't make sense, my response is, "Yes! That's exactly the point! It doesn't make sense!"

Addiction makes people do things that don't make sense. It creates insanity. Why else would people continue to smoke cigarettes knowing that they are going to die because of their addiction? Why else would people continue to drink as they lose family, friends and employment, and as their bodily organs begin to shut down? Why else would people keep going back to engage in immoral, shocking and even dangerous sexual behavior while knowing that it's wrong and may eventually kill them?

This is not to say that every person who commits an immoral sexual act is crazy when he does it. I am talking here about men and women who want to change, who want to stop doing what they're doing, who have tried through prayer, confession, and self-mastery to control their compulsion to do things that are wrong—and then end up going back to them again anyway. This is addiction! It is a disease.

6. We Should Stop Referring to It Only as a Habit or a Problem

Using those words—and avoiding the word "addiction"—minimizes the issue and suggests to everyone that this is just a minor inconvenience that can be adjusted with prayer, positive thinking and self-control. I encourage you to read the essay "Sitting in a Rowboat Throwing Marbles at a Battleship" for a different perspective. This addiction is so much bigger than many of us realize.

7. We Must Quit Thinking That Addicts Can Overcome Addiction On Their Own

Much of the counsel we get in the Church about overcoming the "pornography problem" involves prayer and scripture study, activities we usually undertake on our own and in private. Addiction thrives on isolation. Because of the shame and humiliation associated with the problem and the desire to keep it a secret, the addict will glom onto any suggestion that involves addressing the problem through isolating activities. Addiction loves hearing advice about prayer and scripture study. "More time solo," it says. Obviously, I'm not saying that addicts do away with those two activities. What I am saying, however, is that addicts also need to associate with others who understand addiction because they have personally lived through it and overcome it.

It is our experience that Sexaholics Anonymous (SA) fills this need. In SA, the members encourage and inspire each other to stay sexually sober and to achieve progressive victory over lust. The program works. In my opinion, it works better than any other 12-Step program out there. Its principles are exactly in line with the Restored Gospel. Many LDS men attend these meetings regularly and report that they have achieved a freedom from addiction that had eluded them for years, even decades. Addicts need the help of other recovering addicts to overcome their disease. They cannot do it alone.

We don't need more folks pointing out the supposed problem as if doing so will also solve the problem. We need more people recognizing addictive behavior immediately, and encouraging the addict to get treatment immediately. We need more people understanding that he cannot get over addiction on his own. If a guy with the "little problem" tells us that he has gotten over it on his own, we should be recognizing that he is kidding himself or lying to us (or both) because that's what addicts do. They kid themselves and then lie to others to cover up the addiction. Then they lie again to convince those around them that they've recovered miraculously on their own. Doesn't make sense? Right! It doesn't. Addiction is insanity. It is not a "little problem."

8. We Need to Quit Believing That If They Just Have Enough Faith, Addicts Won't Have to Do the Dirty Work

I once sat in a room of LDS men who were attending a support group for those with a "pornography problem." I was one of the first in the meeting to share my experience of recovery. I talked about going to 12-Step meetings outside the Church several times a week, having a sponsor, making daily phone calls to help others and to help myself stay on the right track, and having increased mental strength and spiritual growth as a result of working through the 12 Steps. I also said I planned to do this for the rest of my life and looked forward to helping other men find recovery like I had.

Many of the participants in that meeting sat open-mouthed, almost stunned, as they listened and contemplated how much time I put into staying in recovery from my addiction every day. When I finished sharing my experience, several of these men immediately clamored to proclaim their colossal faith in the Savior and how they fully expected to be healed or cured (they used the words interchangeably) of their "problem." It was clear that they saw faith in Christ as a shortcut that would save them from the many inconveniences and timewasters to which I was subject. I was, after all, an addict; they just had a "little problem." Remember, as Mormons, we're big on proclaiming that "it is by grace that we are saved, after all we can do." The scripture does not say that "it is by grace that we are saved, after all we can do—except in the limited circumstances of a 'pornography problem,' in which case we line up with the evangelical Christians and just go with the notion of grace alone."

9. We Must Recognize That The Wives of Addicts Need Someone to Talk To—In Addition to a Bishop

Many wives of sex addicts are screaming on the inside. They are confused. They are in pain. This hurts more than anything else they have ever experienced in life. They need to talk with someone who has been there, who has felt and survived the anguish, and who can speak of hope and recovery from the perspective of one who has lived it. Bishops simply cannot provide this insight.

Without hesitation, we recommend S-Anon, a support group for those affected by another's sexual behavior and based on the 12 Steps of Alcoholics Anonymous. I want to be clear about this: These meetings are full of some of the most inspiring, dynamic and beautiful women on the planet. They are helping each other achieve a recovery from the fallout caused by their husbands' behavior that is nothing short of miraculous.

It is not a stopping off place for failed, miserable women before they disintegrate and disappear forever.

When the wife of a sex addict sits down in a bishop's office, one of the first items on his checklist should be to encourage her to begin attending S-Anon meetings. We can give you the phone numbers and e-mail addresses of LDS women who are willing talk about their experience of surviving a sex-addicted husband and how S-Anon helped them return to the land of the living. You can e-mail us at our general e-mail address at *recovery@rowboatandmarbles.org*.

10. We Should Make Sure That Wives Get Information About Sex Addiction

Light and knowledge amount to a death sentence for addiction. Addicts therefore do everything they can to keep their spouses in the dark about their disease and recovery from it. We ought to give every woman in Relief Society a copy of the essay "A Letter to LDS Wives." We should let her know about the recovery website, *RowboatAndMarbles.org*. The site will instill hope and help her know what is really going on inside her husband's brain. The site also has a links page that contains a list of other useful and informative websites geared towards those of the LDS faith.

Dr. Donald L. Hilton, an LDS neurosurgeon, has written a groundbreaking book about recovery from sex addiction entitled *He Restoreth My Soul*. The subtitle says it all: *Understanding and Breaking the Chemical and Spiritual Chains of Pornography Addiction Through the Atonement of Jesus Christ*. The S.A. Lifeline Foundation, a Utah-based non-profit organization that provides information and education about pornography addiction and its impact on individuals, families and society, has published *Understanding Pornography and Sexual Addiction: A Resource for LDS Parents and Leaders* as a guide for rendering help to those now suffering in silence. It fills a critical need among rank and file Church members and leaders by providing them with practical information and recovery tools for assisting addicts and their families in their quest for a solution to their nightmare.

11. We Need to Quit Thinking That We Have to Wait for the Church to Perfect a Program That Will Solve the Problem

That thirteenth Article of Faith of ours is not just window dressing. "If there is anything...of good report or praiseworthy, we seek after these things." Many of us in recovery enthusiastically report that Sexaholics Anonymous (*www.sa.org*) and S-Anon (*sanon.org*) are praiseworthy—and lifesaving. The programs for sexual sobriety and recovery are here with us now and they work!

12. We Must Recognize That There Is Hope for Recovery from Sex and Pornography Addiction

Those of us who have found true sobriety and recovery are living proof.

7. A Letter to Theo

A letter to an LDS guy I sponsored about moral agency and why sponsors are vital to recovery (Theo is not his real name)

DEAR THEO:
Part of a sponsor's job is to offer experience and insight to the guys fighting addiction because the addict who is heavy into his addiction has lost the ability to see clearly. Sometimes the sponsor tells the addict things the addict doesn't want to hear. The addict has to employ some humility, recognize that the sponsor may possess greater knowledge and understanding, and be willing to do what the sponsor suggests.

I'm going to tell you some things about myself and by doing so, I'm hoping you will relate to my situation as it used to be and see the many similarities to your current situation. I have been a working in the professional world since 19XX. I earned a degree from a very competitive East Coast graduate school and then worked for the federal government for a time before taking a job at a big firm in a major city on the West Coast.

I worked long hours, usually going into the office in the dark and coming home in the dark. I resented my bosses. I resented my wife. I resented the government official I had worked for. I resented the graduate school and the professors who didn't give me the grades I felt

I deserved. I resented the firms that didn't make me the job offers I expected. I resented the clients. I resented the other professionals.

At the time, I didn't realize I was so full of resentment. At church I was first the ward mission leader, then the stake mission president. It turns out I also resented the stake missionaries, the bishops and the stake presidency. I resented the people who were taught and converted by the missionaries. In a huge way, I resented the missionaries. Resentment was eating me alive even while I genuinely thought I loved everyone and was generally living a Christ-like life.

I considered myself stronger, smarter and more spiritual than everyone around me. Although I wanted to feel like I was in command, I often felt like I had no control at all over my life because I had to do what so many others wanted me to do. And then I would binge on pornography and masturbation. When I binged, I would tell myself I was doing it because I chose to do it. Although it was unknown to me at the time, I also did it because it made me hurt less emotionally for a little while, and because I felt like I deserved to hurt less.

What I didn't understand was that I was addicted and that my addiction was fabricating reasons, feelings and justifications for acting out. Since I was the smartest, strongest, most spiritual person around, I could only conclude that I was in control and, therefore, that I must be choosing to look at porn. The truth was, however, that I had long since lost my ability to say no to the compulsions to consume pornography and engage in masturbation. *I had no agency.*

As I've read your e-mails, I've noticed that you talk a lot about what people and circumstances around you are "compelling you to do" and how they don't allow you control over your life. Then you describe looking at porn as "expressing your free agency." I think you have got it backwards. A lot of what you're expressing about other people is resentment. While you don't have control over how other people around you behave, you do have control over how you respond to them and your circumstances. You can choose whether to let the resentment continue to seethe inside you, or whether you will do something to get it out of you so you can deal with it. You need to understand that resentment is one of the biggest poisons that trigger addicts to act out, whether with alcohol, cocaine or porn.

About this whole free agency thing, I suggest that you take a fresh look at that kind of thinking. When you (and I'm talking about just you, not anyone else) look at porn, you are *not* "expressing free agency." You have lost your agency. When you look at porn, you are responding to a compulsion that is bigger than you are. You need to see yourself as an alcoholic only instead of being addicted to alcohol, you are addicted to lust.

When your brain demands a hit, you go looking for lust and you satisfy that overwhelming compulsion by looking at porn and engaging in masturbation along with it. That is not free agency. It is the opposite: no agency. Latter-day Saint men who have agency don't look at porn or masturbate. They choose not to do it because, when they think about it, looking at porn and masturbation are insane. A sane person wouldn't engage in that behavior if he had a choice about it.

One of the biggest hurdles for an addict to get over is that first admission that he really is addicted, that he is powerless over his drug and that it will beat him *every time* if he keeps fighting it on his own. Addicts are frequently willing to say they have a "little problem" or that they occasionally have a brief lapse of self control. Addicts minimize the issue. They are usually unwilling to acknowledge to themselves or to anyone else that they are addicted, are powerless and have completely lost control.

That's one of the reasons why sponsors are important. They are recovering addicts themselves. When they look the addict in the eye, they can say, "You are an addict," and they are saying it not in derision, but from the position of those who know because they've been there.

So here's the question for you: Do you believe you are an addict and are powerless over your drug (lust), or do you just think you have a "little problem" with porn? By the way, admitting that you are an addict is not admitting that you are a bad person. It is not admitting that you are a loser, or that you are a failure or that you have no self-control whatsoever. It is not admitting that you are sub-intelligent. It is not admitting that you don't have enough faith in Christ.

When you admit that you are an addict, all you are doing is acknowledging that you are powerless over lust, and that as a result of that powerlessness, your life has become unmanageable. Once you do that, your life actually will change in some amazing ways. You should be excited; things are about to get great.

By the way, if you've read my "Rowboat and Marbles" essay, you've read about my friend with severe depression. She kept praying and praying for Heavenly Father to take away her unhappiness. He did, but He did it through the intermediary of a friend who helped her see what the problem was and see that she needed psychiatric help.

You are in the same position as my friend. For years, you've been praying and asking Heavenly Father to give you strength to overcome your weakness on your own. Heavenly Father has now answered your prayers, but not in the way you expected. He gave you strength to send that first e-mail to *SALifeline.org*. He gave you strength to respond to my e-mails. He has given you a chance to learn, understand, change, heal, recover and be happy. He has given you an opportunity to fix your marriage by first fixing yourself.

As you get more sober and move further into recovery, your wife is going to notice some differences in you. She will see that you're less preoccupied and self-absorbed and that you're more mentally and emotionally present with her and the family. She will notice that you are more interested in spiritual things and more willing to pleasantly take charge of the family's spiritual matters. She will notice a softening in how you treat her. Your kids will notice these changes, too. It's going to be fabulous.

Please make time today to get into the *White Book of Sexaholics Anonymous*. You need to fill your brain with recovery tools that will help you overcome your addictive behavior. I think of it like a big Lego bucket. If you only have two or three Legos in your bucket, they'll rattle around and make a lot of noise, but you won't be able to do much with them. If, on the other hand, you fill your recovery bucket with all the sobriety Legos you can get a hold of, you can then build some very serious recovery. Let me know your thoughts on the reading and give me an answer to the question I asked above.

Talk soon,
Andrew P.

8. The Silent 70 Percent

*Seeing the sex and pornography crisis among
the Latter-day Saints as it really is*

CONSIDER THE FOLLOWING:
- More than 70 percent of men ages 18 to 34 visit a pornography site on the internet in a typical month.
- "We suspect that the LDS community is not any different from the rest of society when it comes to prevalence or magnitude of sexual addictions."
- "The tsunami is coming."

The numbers in the first bullet point above are taken from the statistics page at *SafeFamilies.org*. The quote in the second bullet point is by Dan Gray, a licensed clinical social worker and director of the Life-STAR Network, which specializes in helping Latter-day Saints deal with sexual addictions. He was cited in a series of articles on pornography addiction in the *LDS Church News* in 2007. The quote in the third bullet point is by Todd Olsen, also a licensed clinical social worker and program director of the LifeSTAR network, again in the same Church News series.

If someone asked me to describe how a typical Latter-day Saint might view the "pornography problem" amongst the men in the Church, I would use the numbers 85, 12 and 3. I think a lot of Latter-day Saints would estimate that about 85 percent of male Church members have no problem with pornography. These men may have been exposed to it at some point but have since shunned it as the filth that it is. Our typical Latter-day Saint would also peg the percentage of priesthood holders with a "little pornography problem" at around 12. While this number would be disappointingly high for them, it would acknowledge that pornography is a growing epidemic even among the Saints. That leaves a mere three percent of members who might be considered true addicts, men who (we incorrectly believe) are sadly beyond hope and will struggle through the miserable remainder of their lives before dying and going to hell. In this view of the LDS world, the ranks of the incorrigible are thankfully fairly small.

If this is the perception of the problem in the Church, it is completely off base and is something we must change. As mentioned above, according to *SafeFamilies.org*, 70 percent of men under age 35 look at porn in a typical month. Based on his experience, Dan Gray believes the statistics are roughly the same within the Church as without. What this means then is that possibly 70 percent of the men in a typical elders quorum are looking at porn each month.[1]

The Lord is very clear on the subject of pornography. "And he that looketh upon a woman to lust after her shall deny the faith, and shall not have the Spirit; and if he repents not he shall be cast out" (D&C 42:23). To reinforce the point, the Lord later says that if Melchizedek Priesthood holders look "on a woman to lust after her, or if any shall commit

---

[1] We don't know the exact numbers of Latter-day Saints who regularly consume pornography. We do know that it is a lot. Even if the 70 percent figure is too high by double, this would still mean that approximately one-third of our young adults are getting crushed by the "pornography problem." From the research I have done and from anecdotal experience, both my own and that of others, the 70 percent figure appears to us to be "in the ballpark." Whether you, the reader, accept this number or not, I ask you not to dwell on it too much. The point is that a huge portion of our church population currently suffers directly or indirectly from the effects of the pornography epidemic.

adultery in their hearts, they shall not have the Spirit, but shall deny the faith and shall fear" (D&C 63:16). Elsewhere, the Lord says that a sinner must not only confess but also forsake the sin in order to repent (D&C 58:43). To forsake means "to quit or leave *entirely*; abandon; desert;... to give up or renounce." [See Dictionary.com: *forsake* (my emphasis)].

The individual words in these verses have to mean something. From the Lord's own mouth, those who look at pornography deny the faith and do not have the companionship of the Holy Spirit. If a man returns every couple of months to binge on pornography and masturbation, he has not forsaken the sin, and therefore has not repented of the sin. If the "little problem" could be handled with a quick "I'm really sorry" prayer on the way to the temple for an endowment session, these utterances from the Lord would have no meaning. Neither would verses 36 and 37 of Doctrine and Covenants Section 121:

> [T]he rights of the priesthood are inseparably connected with the powers of heaven, and...the powers of heaven cannot be controlled nor handled *only upon the principles of righteousness*. That they may be conferred upon us, it is true; but when we undertake *to cover our sins*, or to gratify our pride, our vain ambition, or to exercise control or dominion or compulsion upon the souls of the children of men, in any degree of unrighteousness, behold, the heavens withdraw themselves; *the Spirit of the Lord is grieved; and when it is withdrawn, Amen to the priesthood or the authority of that man* [my emphasis].

The 70 percent of men in elders quorums who may regularly be looking at pornography have not forsaken the sin, they are undertaking to cover their sins, and they appear to have disqualified themselves from invoking the power of the priesthood. Through pornography, Satan may have effectively neutralized more than half the priesthood holders in the Church's elders quorums.

We need to understand that the effect of pornography goes way beyond losing the constant companionship of the Holy Ghost. Some of this is tough to hear, which is one of the reasons why I think we don't talk about it very much in the way in which I'm about to tackle it. When the Lord showed the Prophet Joseph Smith and Sidney Rigdon a vision of the three degrees of glory, they described the attributes of their respective citizens. We usually focus on the *celestial* kingdom because, after all, that is where we want to find ourselves and our families. When dealing with the subject of pornography, however, we need to take a hard look at the *telestial* kingdom.

The inhabitants of the telestial kingdom are made up of, among others, liars, adulterers, whoremongers and "whosoever loves and makes a lie" (D&C 76:103). Those LDS men with a "pornography problem" need to pay careful attention here. Addicts are liars. They lie to themselves; they lie to their spouses; they lie to their priesthood leaders; and they try to lie to the Lord. Lying is part of being an addict. One way they try to dodge this reality is by repeatedly telling the big lie: "I am not an addict! I just have a 'little problem.'"

Men who look at pornography necessarily lust after the women on the page or the screen and commit adultery with them in their hearts. They look at one sexually explicit image after another until they have looked at thousands upon thousands of images. They watch one sexually graphic video after another until they have watched thousands upon thousands of videos. Nothing is left to the imagination—and I mean *nothing*. Whether they actually touch another person or not, the distinction becomes irrelevant. They are adulterers.

A whoremonger is frequently described simply as a pimp. Since there are few pimps in the Church, this word doesn't get dissected very often. In fact, a whoremonger is actually "one who consorts with whores; a lecher or pander" (See Dictionary.com: *whoremonger*). Consort means "to associate; keep company" (See Dictionary.com: *consort*). A lecher is "a man given to excessive sexual indulgence; a lascivious [inclined to lustfulness] or licentious [sexually unrestrained] man" (See Dictionary.com: *lecher*). A pander is the pimp mentioned above (See Dictionary.com: *pander*).

The point I'm making is that the term whoremonger encompasses many more individuals than just pimps. A whoremonger is one who keeps company with prostitutes, who is given to excessive sexual indulgence, who is inclined to lustfulness and who is sexually unrestrained.

In my mind, this describes the Mormon man who waits until his wife and children are asleep and then sneaks down to the computer in the family room to spend hours looking at porn and doing what men do when they look at porn.

Finally, I want to look at the other telestial denizen that is often overlooked: he who loves and makes a lie. In "The ABCs of Addiction," I talk about how a man who views pornography *always* ends up objectifying the women around him. I also explain how this objectification extends even to his own wife. She becomes merely one of the objects he uses to satisfy his lust. He may tell her he loves her, but, if he were honest, he would say to her, "You satisfy my lust hunger *almost as well as pornography and masturbation.*" The love he expressed to her across the altar at the temple has become a lie.

Men of the Church who look at porn are lying adulterers who repeatedly engage in whoremonger behavior. They love their wives and make a lie of it. They are indulging in telestial activities. Because they have not forsaken the sin, they have not repented of it. When they die, they will find that their telestial behavior has destined them for telestial glory. As far as I know, there is no divine allowance for the whoremonger behavior of priesthood holders. Their priesthood office is apparently irrelevant. Whoremongers go to hell (D&C 76:84).

"The tsunami is coming." Indeed, it's already here. Like so many other communities of the world, sex and pornography addiction is wiping out the Latter-day Saints. And here we sit, whistling in the wind and trying to convince ourselves that we're adequately addressing the problem. Seventy percent of the elders in our quorums may be consuming pornography and we are not in panic mode about it. Instead, we are talking about increasing temple attendance.[2]

So why aren't we in panic mode? Why does our handling of the "pornography problem" bring to mind Nero fiddling as Rome burned? A big part of the answer has to do with those numbers 85, 12 and 3. In

---

[2] This is not a criticism of the Church's general leadership. They have been warning us from the pulpit for decades about the dangers of pornography. While they have raised the general voice of warning, it has been up to us, the rank and file members of the Church, to understand and implement the warning into our lives. Clearly, we have not done a very good job in the implementation.

the minds of most Latter-day Saints, I think, the majority of us have no problem (the 85 percent), and some of us (the 12 percent) just have a "little problem" that can be fixed with minor improvements to spirituality such as more frequent prayer and scripture study. As for the 3 percent—well, they're too far gone for us to do anything about them, bless their poor, lazy, miserable, sinful, little hearts. Crisis? What crisis? We see three categories of people in the fight against pornography and 97 percent of us are doing great or just have a little problem.

The big surprise is that there are only two groups! There are those with no pornography problem and those with a big pornography problem. There is no middle group! One of the themes throughout my essays is that there is no such thing as a "little problem" when it comes to sex and pornography addiction. Let's return to the 70 percent of the elders quorums who regularly look at pornography. These are the ones with the big problem. They may be addicted, want to stop, but can't. They have tried and tried and tried. Some of them have tried for decades to stop—but they keep going back.

In their minds and in the minds of their local priesthood leaders, it just makes no sense to describe their situation as an addiction. Many of these guys have tremendous faith in the Savior, do their home teaching, fulfill their Church responsibilities (some even serve in leadership roles), attend the temple regularly(!), read their scriptures, hold Family Home Evening, and never under any circumstances do they miss their personal prayers. These guys are spiritual giants! They couldn't possibly be addicts! They are not part of that (imaginary) three percent who rarely attend church, refuse callings, bad-mouth the leadership, and simply *refuse to give up their addiction* as a truly devout Latter-day Saint would! Since most of the "70 percent" don't fit the addict stereotype, we have fabricated a handy category for them: the 12 percent with a "little problem."

We want to believe that if we do all those things that devout Latter-day Saints do, we can't possibly be addicted. It must be something else besides addiction: just a "little problem." And yet, why does anyone die of cancer in this Church of ours? If they do all the things that devout Latter-day Saints do, why doesn't that take care of the cancer? Why does anyone in our Church live an entire lifetime with diabetes? If they do all the things that devout Latter-day Saints do, why doesn't that take care of the diabetes?

The reality is that some devout Mormons die of cancer, some devout Mormons have to live with diabetes—and some devout Mormons have the disease of addiction to sex and pornography. (Please remember King Benjamin's admonition in Mosiah 4:16-22.) We can be addicted to porn and still want to do our home teaching and hold Family Home Evening and say family prayers morning and night and attend the temple(!) and give fabulously insightful talks in sacrament meeting. If we keep returning to our "little problem" it is because our "little problem" is actually an addiction. Left untreated, addiction will steamroll a man's repeated efforts to fortify himself spiritually and overcome his damning behavior. It will overpower him and he will slip up again and again just as he always has—unless he gets help from other people who know how to deal with addiction. There is always hope!

As we've discussed, the "12 percent" may actually consist of about 70 percent of the men under age 35 in the Church. Somehow, they need to come to understand that they may be addicted to sex and pornography; that they can't get over it on their own (as evidenced by the fact that they haven't been able to get over it on their own); that if left untreated, the disease of addiction is progressive and degenerative; and that the disease may eventually progress to a point that it kills them. Before it kills them, however, it will destroy their family, their marriage, their integrity, their faith, their finances, their health and their sanity.

In a way, the disease of sex and pornography addiction has already impaired the sanity of so many of us in the Church. We are viewing the crisis as an insane person would view it. We are responding to it as an insane person would respond to it. We are talking about it as an insane person would talk about it. Over the course of the time I have been in recovery, I have been able to talk with a number of LDS men who are also struggling with or recovering from the "pornography problem" and are in various stages of recovery or non-recovery. Some of those conversations have brought our collective insanity front and center for me.

Several of these LDS guys have been relatively new to the experience and process of 12-Step programs. They were new to the idea of powerlessness over their addiction. The First Step in all the 12-Step programs is that we "admitted that we were powerless over [our addiction], that our lives had become unmanageable." One of the ways that those in long-term recovery help the new guys understand powerlessness is by having them write out on paper a history of their sexual behavior including the pornography and masturbation binges. We then have them write out all of the ways that their behavior has affected their marriage, their family, their service in the Church, their relationships with others, their finances, their education, their employment, and their relationship with God. We have them write out everything they've ever done to try to put a stop to the behavior. We have them write out why these efforts to stop have failed.

We have them write this stuff out on paper so that they don't forget anything and so they have a tangible record of their insanity. Then, when they've finished, we have them read out loud to us what they've written. More often than not, it is a long list. More often than not, it contains more than just pornography and masturbation. When I read my First Step to my sponsor, I sobbed. Until I had to listen to myself make this oral accounting, I had had no idea that my "little problem" had exacted such an enormous toll on me and those around me to the degree it had. Up to that point, my insane brain had compartmentalized and minimized just about everything associated with my addiction.

As I've had that unique experience of listening to other men share their First Step, I always finish with the same series of questions that my sponsor asked me. Many of these men answer with a new humility, filled with a new understanding of their powerlessness, their insanity and the necessity of their absolute reliance on Heavenly Father to do for them what they've been unable to do for themselves. Others, however, have a different reaction that, I think, epitomizes the problem we may have in the Church right now. When I say "problem," I really mean "insanity." We are doing some things that make no sense!

The dialog often goes something like this:

Me: *You've read through a lot of difficult things. I know it was hard on you, but it was also courageous. How do you feel right now?*

Him: *I feel exhausted and very small. I had no idea that all this stuff added up to an addiction. I always thought it was just a "little problem."*

Me: *Do you believe you're addicted to lust?*
Him: *Yes.*
Me: *Do you believe you've been addicted to lust for a long time?*
Him: *Yes.*
Me: *Based on everything you've written out, do you think you're powerless over lust?*
Him: *Absolutely! I am definitely powerless over lust! I've lost every time I've tried to fight it! I just didn't realize it!*
Me: *Do you believe your life has become unmanageable as a result of your powerlessness over lust?*
Him: *Yes, definitely.*
Me: *Do you see how your addiction has progressed, becoming more and more compulsive, more and more demanding, and more and more insane?*
Him: *Yeah, I do. It's scary. I've done things I vowed I'd never do. I've crossed lines I vowed I'd never cross. Little by little I've surrendered to the insanity of my addiction.*
Me: *Do you believe that your disease will eventually progress to the point that it will kill you?*
Him: *Wow. Yeah, I guess I do.*
Me: *Here's my last question: Do you believe that your disease will eventually progress to a point where you will act outside your marriage?*
Him: *[Silence.]*
Me: *[After a pause.] So, do you?*
Him: *No.*
Me: *Why not?*
Him: *Because I would never do that! I would never let it get to that point! I would never let it get that far out of control!*
Me: *I see. Hmm. It looks like we need to talk some more about powerlessness.*

Admitting powerlessness means admitting that we're sitting in a little rowboat with a handful of marbles and our addiction is a battleship steaming straight at us. We are getting crushed time after time. It is hopeless when we fight it on our own. When we truly admit powerlessness, we quickly come to understand that we have to turn it all over to Heavenly Father. He can do for us what we can't do for ourselves.

If I ask that last question and get that final response, it's a pretty strong indicator of whether a guy truly believes he actually is powerless and is willing to admit it. If he doesn't readily admit it, I try to help him see the insanity of his reasoning.

When he insists that his addiction would never progress to a point where he would act outside his marriage, in essence he is admitting, "I am powerless over my addiction *now* and have been powerless for years. No matter how hard I tried, I couldn't get over it. In fact, it's been getting worse. My addiction is progressing, my life is unmanageable and I am going crazy. I can't control it! Nevertheless, *at some point in the future*, when the addiction progresses further, when the compulsions to act out get even stronger, when my life is even more unmanageable—at that point, in some miraculous way, I will then do for myself what I have been unable to do up until now. *Somehow*, I will seize control of my addiction and beat it. Then, I will no longer be powerless over it!" In other words, when things get bad enough, he will suddenly somehow muster enough of his own inner strength to overwhelm and subdue his addiction. That's crazy talk.

Right now, when the problem is "just" pornography and masturbation, he apparently does not have the inner strength to stop doing what he's doing. In the future, however, when the compulsions are pushing him towards webcams, affairs, strip clubs, prostitutes, massage parlors, anonymous sex and the like, he will somehow be able to control those compulsions in a way in which he can't control the "lesser" compulsions right now. Or perhaps he is suggesting that while he doesn't have enough strength to *stop* right now, somehow he does have the strength to keep it from getting *worse* right now. In Harry Potter books, this type of thing is referred to as *magic*.

The fact of the matter is that very few addicted Mormon men are willing to admit that they are powerless over their addiction to lust. They won't even call it an addiction. To them it's just a "little problem." Of course, they believe that God will help them deal with the "little problem," but He will really just provide sort of a spiritual caffeine boost. Heavenly Father will be more of a divine Cheerleader inspiring them as they summon their own strength. These men are going to do the heavy lifting *somehow*. They are going to beat it on their own *somehow*.

The real crisis among Latter-day Saints is not the explosion of addiction to lust facilitated by the internet. The real crisis is how the addicts and those around them are responding to it. Nearly every addict is trying to beat it *on his own* in silence. Local church leaders are encouraging men to keep up the isolating behavior that has failed them in the past and will fail them in the future. A good working definition of true insanity is doing the same failed thing over and over again, hoping for a different result. If personal prayer, scripture study and temple attendance(!) haven't yet caused a full-scale reversal of the crisis of men binging on pornography, masturbation and other sexual behavior, maybe it's time we admit that something is missing from the equation. Why don't we find the LDS men who have achieved long-term recovery from sex and pornography addiction and ask them how they did it? They are out there. They have a story to tell.

Although I've already hit on some very troubling topics, I will end with something that is even more difficult to hear. It has caused me sleepless nights. It has left me baffled and perplexed and wondering if there isn't some way around it. It is based upon the experiences of millions of recovering alcoholics, drug addicts, food addicts, sex addicts, gamblers, shoppers and procrastinators. We who are now in recovery used to be the worst of the worst.

In the early days of Alcoholics Anonymous, many of us had been written off as crazy and locked up in sanitariums or prisons for the criminally insane. Many of us had lost everything. According to doctors and therapists, we were without hope and would die in our disease. We had hit rock bottom.

And then we recovered. We found others like us who were further up the path to sobriety and recovery than we were. We began to associate with them in meetings. We listened to their experiences. We asked them to sponsor us and help us work the steps. We got sober—for real this time—and there were no more slips. We began working to understand and address our character defects. We made lists of the people we had hurt with our behavior and tried to make amends to them. We began to recognize more quickly when we were at fault, then promptly admit it and fix it. We grew closer to Heavenly Father and our fellow human beings, being able to love them for the first time now that our lives had become free of self-absorbed narcissism.

For those of us of the Christian faith, our appreciation for the Atonement of Jesus Christ achieved a new and ever-growing profundity. And through it all, we wanted nothing more than to share what we had found with others. The compulsion to act out with our respective drugs was replaced almost immediately by a near-compulsion to help others learn how to turn things over to Heavenly Father so He could also do for them what they had been unable to do for themselves. As we recovering addicts have come together, we have each experienced an individual miracle as Heavenly Father has changed and healed us.

To our dismay, however, so many others with our same afflictions have come to the edge of the pool, dipped in a big toe and then decided that our swim team requires too much lap work. They're looking for an easier way. After all, they're not really addicted; they just have a "little problem." They are not as bad off as we—the truly sick, truly hopeless addicts—are. And yet, unlike the addicts in recovery, they remain unable to ever find true recovery on their own.

I've talked about this with other recovering addicts. The general consensus based on our collective experiences is this: In order to get sober and into recovery, one must first hit *rock bottom*. Those who have hit bottom become willing to do whatever it takes to get sober. They are willing to do the hard things. Those who have not hit rock bottom, however, are not willing to do whatever it takes. They still believe they have things "under control." They are not ready to turn it over to God because they are still convinced they can do this on their own. They are not ready to surrender. They do not believe they are powerless.

In their *Big Book*, the members of Alcoholics Anonymous have divided alcoholics into four groups. Group 1 is those who are "merely" the heavy drinkers. Group 2 is those who have lost control of the drinking and their behavior. Group 3 is those who have lost jobs, family and integrity, know there is something very wrong with themselves, but still can't stop. Group 4 is those who have lost their minds. They are the dregs of society. They go insane when they drink. Health professionals shake their heads and have little hope for Group 4.

Here's the surprising thing: According to AA, the drinkers that have the greatest likelihood of complete recovery are those in Groups 3 and 4! The guys who are the "furthest gone" are actually the ones who respond best to the 12-Step programs. They get well. They get sober and never drink again! In contrast, the drinkers who disappoint the most are those in Groups 1 and 2. They think they're still in control. They often still enjoy being drunk. They are some of the ones who have not hit rock bottom. They are not willing to do whatever it takes. They do not recover. Apparently, they need to "fall" to Groups 3 or 4 before they get serious about recovery.

Sex addicts, in my opinion, are the same. The guys in Group 1 think their "little pornography problem" is not even a problem. Group 2 is the sex addicts who think they may possibly have a "little pornography problem," but it's nothing that they can't handle on their own in isolation. They are still "in control." Group 3 prefers the company of the porn on the computer to real people. They have begun to isolate in earnest. They know they have a serious problem but can't stop. Their acting out is more frequent than binging and they may have begun acting out with other people. Their fantasy has overrun their reality. They're miserable and scared most of the time. They don't know what to do. For Group 4, sex is the focus of their lives. They think they'll die without it and they feel like they're going to die even if they try to slow down. Their addiction to sex has made them crazy. It has destroyed their lives. These are the folks that we would have pigeon-holed in the "3 percent."

Those in Groups 3 and 4 are the ones who jump into the 12-Step programs with vigor. They have far less trouble admitting that they are powerless because they have clearly experienced it and recognize it. They want to get well. They are willing to do whatever it takes. Most of the addicts in the "70 percent" in the Church, however, are in Groups 1 and 2. They have not yet hit rock bottom. They think they're still in control. They do not believe they are powerless. They are not yet willing to do whatever it takes. They are not finding sobriety. They are isolating and continuing to act out. They binge in secret and tell themselves it's not really that big of a deal. They still believe they'll be able stop before it gets worse. Their local priesthood leaders unwittingly mislead them by offering affirmations that they're still in control and that they can stop on their own if they just understand the nature of their sins, if they just keep in their minds the adoring faces of their wife and children, or *if they really want to.*

I would like to think there's some way for the men in Groups 1 and 2 to get into recovery earlier in the addiction process. Unfortunately, if history is any indicator of future outcomes, the men of Groups 1 and 2 will have to hit their own rock bottom in their own time before they can get well. They will have to get worse before they can get better. No one can hit bottom for them—not their wives, not their families, not their priesthood leaders. That's the big dilemma that I can't figure out. I don't want to admit that this is the way it has to be, but I can't find any other way of looking at it. I can't find anyone who has had a different experience.

Many of the unrecovered addicts who read this will do what they've always done. They'll dismiss what I'm saying because they believe they are stronger, smarter and more spiritual than I and the other "real addicts" are. We "real addicts" are weak, they say, so we have to do things the weak way. The unrecovered addicts, on the other hand, have practically enough faith in Jesus Christ to be translated—at least that's how they see it in their own minds. With faith as massive as theirs, they won't have to do the dirty work. Of course, complete denial of reality is a hallmark of addiction, especially for those in Groups 1 and 2.

So what's the answer? Sex and pornography addicts in the Church need to come to terms with their powerlessness. They need to acquire and employ some humility—even if there's a cost associated with it. This can best be done by finding and talking to one of those addicts in long-term recovery about why he no longer acts out on his addiction. If a recovering sex addict can't be located, a recovering alcoholic will be able to tell practically the same story.

Nothing will lead an addict to true recovery more surely than associating with recovering addicts. Quote me on that. Print it out and tape it to the computer monitor and the bathroom mirror and the dashboard of your car. If you want to see the miraculous power of the Atonement at work, talk to a recovering addict. Listen to what humility sounds like. Learn about powerlessness and how to truly surrender to God. Doing this truly will require an act of humility on your own part. It will require the addicts among the "70 percent" to utter those horrifying words, "Maybe I can't do this on my own. Maybe I need other people to help me."

Another part of the answer is that those surrounding sex and pornography addicts need to quit enabling the addicts. So many wives are understandably in pain from the damage caused by their husbands' addictive behavior. But they, too, don't want to admit that this is anything more than a "little problem." "If he really loved me," they say, "he'd just stop doing this!" These wives should be assured that in nearly all cases, their husband really does love them. The husband's addiction, however, doesn't love these wives—at all. It loves only itself. It just wants to keep feeding on lust, whatever the cost to the wife, the husband and everyone around them. These husbands are in little rowboats and they each have a handful of marbles. Their addiction is a battleship. No one can sink a battleship with marbles—not even the strongest, smartest, most spiritual guy on the planet.

These men need help, and they need it from people who have experience treating and overcoming sex and pornography addiction. This means professional counselors, sponsors and 12-Step support groups. If the wives and the bishops do not have that recovery experience, their ability to help the addicts will be extremely limited. They need to understand that these men have a real disease called *addiction*. They cannot simply *get* well by *being* well. Fortunately, they can get well—if they become willing to do *whatever it takes*.

I suppose my message here is that we should be in crisis mode. Seventy percent of the men in our elders quorums may regularly be looking at pornography. Most of them are trying to stop and yet they can't. They think it's just a "little problem" because men of their spiritual stature don't have addictions. They think that prayer, scripture study and temple attendance(!) will someday *somehow* eradicate their "little problem" even though this "treatment plan" hasn't worked in the past for more than a few months. They don't understand that their "treatment plan" is actually denial, dishonesty and isolation hard at work keeping them from getting the help they need from others to overcome their addiction. They don't recognize that their addiction is progressively getting worse. They don't see that they are crossing lines they vowed they'd never cross. They are sitting alone in tiny rowboats throwing marbles at battleships. They are losing the war.

At the beginning of the Second World War, Germany invaded Poland. Using a strategy called blitzkrieg or "lightning war," the Germans sent fast-moving tanks deep into Poland to overwhelm the defending forces. In response, the Poles called up their cavalry—on horses! They sent soldiers on horses because that's all they had. The Polish cavalry was of course annihilated. There could have been no other outcome when men on horses went up against tanks.

Satan has an army of tanks laying down a barrage of deadly filth in the form of pornography and licentious sexual behavior in our society. These tanks have invaded the homes of even the most devout Latter-day Saints. They are wiping us out. And we are sending out many of our best men to fight Satan's tanks—on horses! As one man after another is blown from his saddle, we seem surprised. How could this be happening? How could we be losing if God is on our side?

Heavenly Father even has a fleet of nuclear-powered tanks of His own. Oddly, though, it is sitting unused, off to the side, practically hidden and forgotten. It is dismissed by Church leaders and members alike as irrelevant and unreliable. Here's why: Those driving the tanks are *recovering sex and pornography addicts*. We used to act out on our addiction, but now we have stopped—permanently.

Like no one else, we, the recovering sex and pornography addicts, know those tanks. We know how to take them apart and put them back together. We know how to drive them. We know the roads, we know the ditches, we know the forests and the fields, and we know the mountains and the deserts—because we've been there. We know how to disrupt and overcome the addiction because we've done it. We understand the enemy as no one else can because we've lived under his tyranny for years—and then we escaped with the help of other recovering addicts.

We have a story to tell. It is a story of recovery, hope and redemption. It is a story that the 70 percent—and all those around them—need to hear. Find us. We are ready to tell our story. We are ready to turn the tide. Our story begins and ends with these words:

RECOVERY IS POSSIBLE AND IT IS WONDERFUL!

9. Is Recovery Even Possible?

The short answer is a resounding YES!

THE LONGER ANSWER is that you can recover from sex addiction and never act out again—if you do what is necessary to achieve sexual sobriety. Addiction is a disease—a treatable disease. In order to treat it, however, you must, in my opinion, get past the idea that you will be cured if you just pray hard enough. I prayed for 36 years to be cured. Finally, I heard a quiet voice in my heart and mind whisper that I needed to quit relying solely on prayer and start *doing* something so the Lord could then do His part. He did not let me down.

It turns out that addiction is not just a spiritual malady. There are physical and emotional components as well. In much the same way that we need to treat and regulate diabetes, we need to treat and regulate addiction. When I was acting out on my addiction, I was unconsciously trying to self-medicate to dull the pain in my heart and mind that was originally the result of depression and childhood sexual and emotional abuse. As a child, I had learned to disappear into fantasy where all the women were nice to me and happy to see me. As I grew older, the fantasies grew more complex and more sexual, fueled by occasional binges of pornography. Fantasy was my mind's coping mechanism. I learned it as a child; I perfected it as an adult.

If you cannot stop looking at pornography or engaging in other sexual behavior that you think is wrong, you need to consider the possibility that you are not merely listening to the naughty voice of a little red devil with a pitchfork on your shoulder telling you to do dirty things. There is a distinct possibility that, like me, you have developed a lust and fantasy coping mechanism that "helps" you deal with the unhappy and stressful times in your life.

You also need to understand that there is a difference between *sin* and *addiction*, and a difference between *repentance* and *recovery*. Addiction is not sin; repentance is not recovery. They are all interconnected, but they are not the same thing. Sex addiction compels you to sin, but it is not the same thing as sin. Likewise, just because you repent of your sins, it does *not* automatically mean that you have recovered from your sex addiction.

Think about it. You have sincerely repented so many times that you can't count them anymore. Why then do you keep going back to the pornography and acting out sexually? Is it because your repentance isn't sincere enough? Do you not cry hard enough? Do you not have enough resolve or conviction or contrition? Maybe it's something else. Is it possible that the issue is not a lack of *repentance from sin*, but rather a lack of *recovery from addiction*?

So what do you do to find recovery? The first thing you have to do is get in contact with someone who has suffered from, but is successfully overcoming, sex addiction. You need to talk to someone who has been to hell and lived to tell about it. You need to talk to someone who can look you in the eye and tell you flat out, "I know what you've been through because I have been there myself. I can help you get better. You can watch me and do what I do. You can ask me questions and I will tell you the answers from experience." In 12-Step programs we call this guy a sponsor. He will save your life. We will help you find one if you e-mail us at *recovery@rowboatandmarbles.org*.

In addition, you need to connect with a 12-Step group. You need the fellowship of those who have gone before you and found recovery. Contrary to what the ignorant and self-righteous might believe, such groups are full of people who have humbly and successfully found real sexual sobriety and are sharing their experience, strength and hope with others who want to do the same. They are some of the most extraordinary individuals I have ever met. The meetings are positive, inspiring and hopeful because of those people who are in recovery.

Your addiction wants you to remain alone—solitary, unhappy and cut off from people who can help you. Addiction thrives on loneliness, shame and despair. If you want to deal with your addiction in a way that works, walk into a 12-Step meeting and make some friends. I promise they will greet you with smiles.

Finally, to recover, you need to heal up the wounds that cause the pain you are trying to medicate. A therapist or professional counselor can help you understand what is going on that makes you hurt. The Lord wants you to be whole—spiritually, mentally and physically. I am sure of that.

If I can instill one idea in your head, it is this: *You can definitely recover—but you cannot recover on your own*! By contrast, you most definitely can stay addicted on your own. As I said, your addiction's continued survival depends on your remaining isolated. Like me, you've proven ten thousand times that going solo is a perfect recipe for failure. Even if you're the toughest, smartest, most spiritual person you know, rest assured that your addiction is more cunning, baffling and powerful than you are—and it doesn't care a bit about your strength of spirit. Reach out to those who have gone before you. It will save your life; it will save your soul.

Recovery and sexual sobriety feel fabulous! Please let those in recovery share their experience, strength and hope with you.

10. This is What Recovery Feels Like!

Ever wonder what goes on in the mind of a recovering sex addict? Read this!

I AM A GRATEFULLY RECOVERING sex and pornography addict. As a result of sex abuse by a neighbor, exposure to pornography by the same neighbor and emotional abuse at home during my childhood, I became a sex addict at the age of six and have been fighting for my life and sanity ever since.

Along with many others, I was under the false impression that my addiction was really just a "little problem" that more faith and a simple attitude adjustment could fix—eventually. As my addiction grew and became progressively more dangerous and out of control, however, I eventually resigned myself to the belief that I was destined for hell and could only hope to live out the remainder of my miserable life as best I could. Unable to find anything that really worked or anyone who could really help, I felt my only option was to continue fighting my battle in secret while doing all I could to be a good husband and father to the extent possible.

The compartmentalizing of my life into the "real" and the "secret" was debilitating on every front: mentally, emotionally, physically and spiritually. I finally reached a point where I simply could not go on. I broke.

In early 2010, over 35 years after the nightmare began, a friend in another state talked to me on the phone and introduced me to Sexaholics Anonymous. The result has been the complete sexual sobriety I had sought for decades but failed to find. It saved my marriage and my life.

I quickly learned that sexual sobriety and recovery elude so many of us addicts because we do not understand that our addiction is so much bigger, stronger and more cunning than we are. As I was writing about my recovery experience one day, the vision came to my mind of a six-year-old boy sitting in a little rowboat with a handful of marbles. A grey battleship was headed straight towards him and was going to crush him. In desperation, the boy was heaving the marbles at the ship as hard as he could, trying to sink it.

This pathetic picture of a frightened child frantically throwing marbles at a battleship finally and accurately captured the sheer futility of 35 years of fighting a battle I could not win and was ill-equipped even to undertake. Thus, the name of our website was born.

The very first thing I learned in recovery was that I had lost the war, or more precisely, every single battle I ever engaged in, because I did not understand that my addiction truly was more powerful than I was. When I fought it, it fought back with ten times more ferocity. I simply could not win. I could only surrender—not to the addiction, mind you, but to God. It was in surrendering, however, that I found victory.

In Sexaholics Anonymous, we work through the 12 Steps of recovery as originally outlined in Alcoholics Anonymous. The first step is that we "admitted that we were powerless over lust [and] that our lives had become unmanageable." It took surrender for me to understand and acknowledge that I truly was powerless over my sex addiction and that it was progressing to the point where it would soon kill me. And that's when my surrender began killing the obsession!

Following in short order for me was the second of the 12 Steps, when I came "to believe that [God] could restore [me] to sanity." As a man of faith, I had always assumed that my life was guided by my faith. Imagine my shock when I discovered that I was, in fact, trying to "save myself on my own terms" all while professing my faith and acceptance of Christ and His infinite Atonement.

Without realizing it, I had been crying out for the Lord to save me not so much from my addiction, but from the necessity of doing everything I could on my end so that He could then save me on His end. I really wanted Him to save me—from doing the dirty work. Poof! I'm cured! Fortunately, it doesn't work that way.

I have the privilege of working through the program of recovery in Sexaholics Anonymous with some of the greatest souls I have ever encountered. As we recovering addicts have journeyed together, buoying each other up as we move forward, my soul and mind and heart have changed. God has performed a miracle in my life. He has made the blind see; he has healed the leper; he has forgiven the sinner.

My prayers are different now. In the past, my prayers of repentance were desperate. I cried out for forgiveness and then for the strength to continue the bitter and bloody fight with an unrelenting enemy. Now my prayers of repentance are prayers of gratitude. I thank the Lord for sending one angel after another to help me find a solution, a sobriety and a recovery from an addiction that was destroying me. With a quiet confidence I can now ask God to accept my offering of a broken heart and contrite spirit as demonstrated by the fact that I have finally been able to forsake my sins, something I had tried and failed to do for more than a third of a century.

I am not cured. I will always be an addict. As I've said in meetings, "I am sober and in recovery, but I'm always about fifteen minutes away from acting out on my addiction." I say this to remind myself and others that recovery is a journey not a destination. If I stop working my program and stop trying to share the message of recovery from addiction with others, I am certain to fall again. I don't intend to let that happen.

Like Alma, I wish I were an angel. I want to cry out to the entire world that there is an escape from the deadly grip of sex and pornography addiction. The Lord has described our modern day as one in which people's iniquities would be "spoken from the housetops." As the internet has come to permeate nearly every facet of our modern lives and very little remains secret, I have often thought that this is surely what He had in mind.

In a way, the internet is allowing me to meld Alma's prayer with the Lord's description of modern life in what will hopefully be a successful undertaking to save lives, marriages and, ultimately, the souls of some of God's children. As my sins are "spoken from the housetops" by means of an electronic megaphone, I pray that the message reaches the ears, eyes and hearts of those who are suffering in confusion and silence, as the voice of an angel crying out that...

Recovery is possible and it is wonderful!

Notes

NOTES

Notes

Notes

NOTES

NOTES

Notes